Lecture Notes on
Forensic Medicine

To Eileen and Jean

Lecture Notes on Forensic Medicine

DAVID J. GEE
CBE, MB, BS, FRCPath, DMJ
Emeritus Professor of Forensic Medicine
University of Leeds

ALAN A. WATSON
JP, MA, MB, BS, FRCP, FRCPath, DMJ, DTM&H
Regius Professor of Forensic Medicine
University of Glasgow

FIFTH EDITION

BLACKWELL SCIENTIFIC PUBLICATIONS

OXFORD LONDON

EDINBURGH BOSTON MELBOURNE

©1968, 1975, 1979, 1984, 1989 by
Blackwell Scientific Publications
Editorial offices:
Osney Mead, Oxford OX2 0EL
8 John Street, London WC1N 2ES
23 Ainslie Place, Edinburgh EH3 6AJ
3 Cambridge Center, Suite 208
   Cambridge, Massachusetts 02142, USA
107 Barry Street, Carlton
   Victoria 3053, Australia

First published 1968
Second edition 1975
Third edition 1979
Fourth edition 1984
Reprinted 1986
Fifth edition 1989

Set by Time Graphics, Singapore
and printed and bound
in Great Britain by Billing and Sons Ltd,
Worcester

DISTRIBUTORS

Marston Book Services Ltd
PO Box 87
Oxford OX2 0DT
(*Orders*: Tel: (0865) 791155
          Fax: (0865) 791927
          Telex: 837515)

USA
Year Book Medical Publishers
200 North LaSalle Street
Chicago, Illinois 60601
(*Orders*: Tel: (312) 726-9733)

Canada
The C.V. Mosby Company
5240 Finch Avenue East
Scarborough, Ontario
(*Orders*: Tel: (416) 298-1588)

Australia
Blackwell Scientific Publicatons
(Australia) Pty Ltd
107 Barry Street
Carlton, Victoria 3053
(*Orders*: Tel: (03) 347-0300)

British Library
Cataloguing in Publications Data

Gee, D.J. (David John)
   Lecture notes on forensic medicine. —
   5th ed.
   1. Forensic medicine
   I. Title   II. Watson, A.A.
   614′.1

   ISBN 0-632-02595-6

Contents

Introduction

This book is intended to provide the undergraduate with an account of the basic principles of the subject so as to equip him or her with sufficient knowledge to be able to recognise and cope with minor medico-legal problems arising in his or her practice and to appreciate when further information and specialised assistance is needed. Detail, therefore, especially in the field of toxicology, is omitted. Further information can be obtained from any of the textbooks listed on p. 221. We are grateful for the opinions of the reviewers of the previous editions, and hope that we have profited from their advice.

In the last edition it was felt that there was a lack of sufficient information on the Scottish aspects of law and practice. Hence the joint authorship of this edition. We hope that it remedies the deficiency.

As always, we are grateful to our teachers; to our colleagues for all their assistances; and to our wives for their unfailing support.

David J. Gee
Alan A. Watson

Part 1
Medico-Legal Aspects of Medical Practice

Chapter 1
The Medical Profession and the General Medical Council

A member of the medical profession has been trained in the practice of medicine, has demonstrated his competence by passing a qualifying examination, and is bound by a code of conduct to protect the interests of his patients. Therefore it is necessary that members of the public may be able to distinguish a practitioner with these qualifications from an unqualified person who, although practising medicine, has not received such a training and is not bound by any code of conduct.

Up to 1858 there were no satisfactory means by which a person in need of medical attention could make such a distinction. The first attempt was made during the reign of Henry VIII by an Act of Parliament which put control of the profession into the hands of the Royal College of Physicians, and gave the College powers to prosecute unqualified practitioners. This failed to suppress quacks.

The main statutory regulations establishing the medical profession were made in the nineteenth century. The most important Acts are:

Medical Act 1858

This Act had the stated object of distinguishing qualified from unqualified medical practitioners. A governing body for the profession, the General Council, was established, with duties to compile and maintain a Medical Register, to supervise medical education, and to exercise disciplinary functions. At this time practitioners could qualify for inclusion in the Register on grounds of experience, even though not possessing qualifying diplomas. Penalties were incurred by persons falsely pretending to be registered.

Medical Act 1886

This made possession of a qualifying degree or diploma obligatory before registration. The General Council was made responsible for maintaining the standard of such qualifying examinations. Provision was made for election of some members of the Council by the registered practitioners; previously the Council had only consisted of persons nominated by the Crown, and representatives of the various licensing bodies, i.e. the Colleges and Universities granting degrees or diplomas recognised as registrable qualifications. The Act also made provision for the recognition of medical qualifications of Colonial (now Commonwealth) countries.

Medical Act 1950

The Act made a period of postgraduate training under supervision compulsory, during which time the practitioner is provisionally registered. Proof of having completed such training satisfactorily is necessary before full registration. The General Medical Council (GMC) became officially so called, and a committee of its members, called the Disciplinary Committee, was formed to enquire into alleged instances of unprofessional conduct, a function which had previously been exercised by the whole Council. The maximum penalty for falsely purporting to be a fully registered medical practitioner was raised by this Act to £500.

Medical Act 1956

This amended and consolidated the previous statutes.

Medical Act 1969

Various modifications of the register were introduced, with two lists of registered persons, the *principal* list, and the *overseas* list, and with a separate register for *temporarily* registered doctors. Provisionally registered, Commonwealth and foreign practitioners are to be indicated in the register. In addition to the initial registration fee, the GMC was empowered to charge an annual retention fee. The term 'serious professional misconduct' replaced 'infamous conduct', and the GMC could suspend a doctor's registration as an alternative to erasure.

Medical Act 1978

The Act increased the proportion of elected members of the Council. Advice on professional conduct or medical ethics could be given by the Council and members of the profession. Three committees of the Council were established, the Preliminary Proceedings Committee, the Professional Conduct Committee and the Health Committee. Modifications were made to the procedure of dealing with disciplinary cases, and arrangements were made for dealing with a doctor who was unfit to practise due to illness. An Education Committee was established. The term 'limited registration' replaced 'temporary registration', with different requirements.

Medical Act 1983

This act consolidated and repealed the 1956, 1969, and 1978 Acts. It embodies their provisions and is the principal Act at present. Its new provisions are largely concerned with implementing regulations in connection with the EEC.

General Medical Council

The constitution of the General Medical Council (GMC) is constituted by

Order in Council. At present the GMC consists of 50 members elected by the profession, 34 appointed by licensing bodies (e.g. the Royal College and Universities) and 13 nominated by the Crown. There are four statutory committees: Education, Preliminary Proceedings, Professional Conduct and Health.

Functions

Education

The Education Committee has the responsibility for determining the standard of medical education and examinations and of supervising the provision of training in the pre-registration period. Inspection of examinations and of courses is carried out by inspectors and by visitors appointed by the Committee.

The Medical Register

This is compiled by the Registrar of the Council and is published annually. It contains the names, qualifications, dates of registration and addresses of all provisionally and fully registered medical practitioners. The qualifying degree or diploma and various approved additional qualifications, including qualifications granted by member states of the EEC, may be registered. The entry in the Medical Register is accepted by the Courts as proof of the doctor's status. Provisionally registered practitioners are indicated by an asterisk (*).

There are additional lists, which are not normally published; an overseas list of registered doctors residing overseas; a visiting overseas doctors list; and a visiting EEC practitioners list.

There is an additional register, the register of medical practitioners with limited registration. Such a practitioner is one who has been selected for work in the United Kingdom in a post approved by the GMC. He must have an acceptable overseas qualification, a knowledge of English, and have a good character and the necessary skill and experience. He must have passed, or been exempted from the PLAB test (the test of knowledge of English and of professional knowledge and competence conducted by the Professional and Linguistic Assessments Board). His employment must be supervised by a fully registered doctor.

Doctors from member states of the EEC may work in the United Kingdom without prior registration with the GMC, but have to provide the Registrar with a declaration of recognised qualifications and of the fact that they are lawfully practising medicine in a member state.

Registration allows the doctor certain privileges. He is entitled to use the description 'registered', or 'duly qualified medical practitioner'. He may hold appointments in most hospitals and public services, practise within the

National Health Service (NHS), issue certain statutory certificates, such as death certificates, and prescribe controlled drugs. He can sue for fees unless he is a Fellow of the Royal College of Physicians. He may be exempted on application from jury service. Provisional registration restricts the doctor to practise within hospital in certain approved training posts, but within these posts he may practise as though fully registered.

The Medical Register is kept up to date by means of periodic enquiries by post to registered practitioners, asking them to confirm that the entry under their names in the Register is correct, e.g. that there has been no change of address.

Removal of a practitioner's name from the Register may occur in certain circumstances:

1 On the death of the practitioner. This event will be notified to the GMC by the Registrar of Births and Deaths.
2 Penal erasure (see below).
3 Failure to reply to the Registrar's enquiry.
4 Failure to pay the annual retention fee.
5 Entries made by error or fraud.
6 On the request of the practitioner, at the discretion of the GMC.

Health Committee

This committee was set up under the Act to consider cases where a practitioner's fitness to practise is seriously impaired by reason of his physical or mental condition.

The procedure is designed to try to avoid action by the Committee itself if possible. When information is received by the GMC that a doctor is sufficiently ill for his work to be affected, this is first considered by the President, or by another member called the Preliminary Screener. If the information appears to merit further enquiry, the doctor is informed and invited to undergo examination by two medical examiners. The Preliminary Screener informs the doctor of their recommendations for treatment and any restrictions on his practice, and if he accepts, and abides by their recommendations no further action is taken.

If, however, the doctor rejects the recommendations or fails to follow them, the Preliminary Screener refers the case to the Health Committee, which consists of 12 members, one being non-medical, together with legal and medical assessors. Cases may also be referred to the Health Committee by the Preliminary Proceedings or the Professional Conduct Committee. The Health Committee may suspend the doctor's registration for a period not exceeding 12 months; or make his registration conditional on his complying with directions of the Committee designed to protect his interests, or those of the public, for a period of up to 3 years.

The principal type of condition likely to be dealt with by the Health Committee is mental illness, possibly associated with alcoholism or drug addiction.

Discipline

By law the GMC is given disciplinary jurisdiction over registered medical practitioners, but only to the extent of deciding whether a doctor has been guilty of conduct which renders him unfit to remain a member of the profession. Therefore the only punitive action which the Council may take is to remove the name of the doctor from the Medical Register, thereby indicating that he is no longer a member of the profession, or to modify his registration for a time. It does not impose fines or other forms of punishment.

Circumstances leading to disciplinary enquiry

1 *Conviction of a statutory offence.* The conviction of a doctor of any offence in a Criminal court in the British Isles, whether grave, e.g. rape, or trivial, e.g. a drinking offence, is automatically notified to the GMC by the Clerk of the Court, or the police. The finding of adultery by a doctor in a Matrimonial Court will also be notified.

2 *Accusation of serious professional misconduct* (this term has replaced the older form 'infamous conduct'). Such a complaint may be brought by a member of the public or a fellow-practitioner or a person acting in a public capacity. The allegation concerns conduct which is not a statutory offence, but may constitute a breach of medical ethics.

A definition of infamous conduct was given by Lopes, L.J. in 1894, 'If a medical man in the pursuit of his profession has done something with regard to it which would be reasonably regarded as disgraceful or dishonourable by his professional brethren of good repute and competency, then it is open to the GMC, if that be shown, to say that he has been guilty of infamous conduct in a professional respect.'

Examples of serious professional misconduct

A comprehensive list of types of behaviour which would constitute serious professional misconduct does not exist. However, under the recent legislation the GMC is empowered to provide advice for the profession on standards of professional conduct, or on medical ethics. For this purpose the Standards Committee has been formed.

In an examination emergency the student would probably be able to remember the oft-quoted five As:

1 Abortion.
2 Adultery.

3 Advertising.

4 Addiction.

5 Association.

The GMC issues a pamphlet, the 'Blue Book', called *Professional Conduct and Discipline: Fitness to Practise*. It should be consulted for full details. The following abbreviated list only indicates the main varieties of conduct liable to lead to disciplinary action.

Disregard of professional responsibilities to patients

Gross negligence in diagnosis or treatment. The subject of negligence is dealt with in Chapter 6. To constitute serious professional misconduct the doctor's actions would have to go beyond the sphere of ordinary negligence on one occasion, even though that would render the doctor liable to civil action, and would have to consist of persistent and gross neglect of his patients' interests by failing to apply accepted methods of diagnosis and treatment, as a result of which the patients were harmed. Persistent failure to attend patients through idleness or carelessness would constitute such conduct.

Improper delegation of duties — covering. A doctor has to ensure proper delegation of professional duties, and that junior colleagues are competent to deal with the delegated duties. The same considerations apply to delegation to nursing staff. Covering means associating with unregistered medical practitioners in such a way that members of the public are misled as to their true status. Thus, by administering anaesthetics to enable such a practitioner to perform operations, the doctor might cause patients to believe that the operator himself was a member of the medical profession, or that his methods had received general approval by the profession. Allowing such a person to use the doctor's premises, staff, or instruments might have the same effect.

Abuse of doctor's knowledge, skill or privileges

Illegal abortion. This is one of the most heinous of all medical sins, and a doctor who is shown to have been guilty of such action is almost certain to be 'struck off'. Therefore it is particularly important that a doctor should avoid even suspicion of this offence. If he is consulted by a pregnant woman, and there appears to him to be adequate medical reasons, physical or psychological, for the termination of the pregnancy, he should always refer the case to recognised specialists in the relevant fields of medicine, and obtain their opinions, before embarking on any course of action (see section on therapeutic abortion, Chapter 4).

Moreover, he should be scrupulously careful to avoid being implicated unknowingly in the procuring of an abortion. He should be quite sure of the nature of any minor gynaecological operation or procedure at which he is asked to assist, or administer an anaesthetic.

He should also be very wary of performing a gynaecological examination in his surgery, when witnesses are absent, on a woman of child-bearing age, lest she be pregnant, and having subsequently aborted, accuses him of being responsible. Indeed, if the woman should die of some complication of the abortion, he might be charged with manslaughter.

Improper use of controlled drugs. This means the use of drugs to produce or gratify addiction, either of the doctor or his patient. It also covers the commission of offences, contrary to the Misuse of Drugs Act, for instance the purveying of such drugs to unauthorised persons.

Therefore it again behoves the doctor to avoid any possible suspicion by understanding and adhering strictly to the relevant law, e.g. by ensuring that his supplies of controlled drugs are accurately accounted for. He should be especially cautious when prescribing drugs of addiction, particularly to young people with non-fatal illnesses, and to temporary patients who may be addicts, using a story of absence from their usual medical practitioner as a means of obtaining supplies of drugs; overprescription must be avoided, and drugs not used by a patient must be retrieved and destroyed, lest they be disposed of to unauthorised persons.

False or misleading certificates. As the number of forms or certificates to be completed during the course of medical practice continues to increase, so does the risk that a doctor, from overwork or carelessness, will be tempted to issue them without ensuring that the information he gives is accurate. But he does this at his peril. To issue a National Insurance Certificate without seeing the patient, or to complete cremation form C while confined to bed by illness, without having seen the body or the doctor issuing form B, is to invite criticism, or worse, disciplinary proceedings, and deliberate falsification of certificates is a very serious offence.

Abuse of the doctor–patient relationship

Adultery or improper conduct or association with a person with whom the doctor has a professional relationship constitutes serious professional misconduct.

The professional relationship may be obvious, as when the person concerned is the doctor's patient or less immediately apparent as when the person is a relation of a patient. The important point is that the doctor made the acquaintance of the person as the result of his professional services, and that the adultery or improper association commenced while the professional relationship existed, even though it was subsequently severed.

An improper relationship may exist, short of actual adultery. Thus the following comments were made by the Judicial Committee of the Privy Council when upholding a decision of the GMC: 'A doctor gains entry to the home in the trust that he will take care of the physical and mental health of the family. He must not abuse his professional position so as, by act or word, to impair in the least the confidence and security which should subsist between husband and wife. His association with the wife becomes improper when by look, touch, or gesture he shows undue affection for her, when he seeks opportunities of meeting her alone, or does anything else to show that he thinks more of her than he should. Even if she sets her cap at him, he must in no way respond or encourage her. If she seeks opportunities of meeting him, which are not necessary for professional reasons, he must be on his guard. He must shun any association with her altogether, rather than let it become improper. He must be above suspicion.'

'It was suggested that a doctor, who started as the family doctor might be in a different position when he became a family friend. His conduct on social occasions was to be regarded differently from his conduct on professional occasions. There must, it was said, be cogent evidence to show that he abused his professional relationship. This looks very like a suggestion that he might do in the drawing-room that which he might not do in the surgery. No such distinction can be permitted. A medical man who gains the entry into the family confidence by virtue of his professional position must maintain the same high standard when he becomes the family friend.'

Improper disclosure of confidential information. The matter is discussed in Chapter 7. Briefly, a doctor should normally keep secret any information obtained about his patients, and only divulge it on direction of a Judge in a Court of Law. On the occasions when it becomes necessary, in the interests of the community, for the doctor to disclose knowledge obtained in confidence, he must observe the rules of privileged communication.

Conduct discreditable to the doctor, or to the profession

Evidence, such as notification of conviction, that a doctor has been guilty of such offences as fraud, forgery, theft , etc.

Alcoholism and drug addiction. A doctor who suffers from either of these conditions may be a danger to his patients, and therefore unfit to continue in practice. However, they are curable, so when a complaint or a notification of conviction is received for the first time in respect of a particular doctor, the Professional Conduct Committee may postpone its decision in order to allow the doctor time to undergo treatment, or refer the case to the Health Committee. Nevertheless alcoholism or drug addiction constitutes serious professional misconduct, and repeated complaints or notifications of conviction, e.g. for drunken driving will result in penal erasure.

Abuse of financial opportunities. Examples of such abuse are:

1 Improperly obtaining money by demanding fees from Health Service patients when they are entitled under the National Health Service Acts to free treatment.

2 Commercialisation of a secret remedy.

3 Dichotomy or 'fee-splitting' as when part of a private patient's fee is handed by a specialist to the general practitioner as a reward for having referred the patient to him.

4 Prescribing drugs or appliances in which the practitioner has a financial interest. This, of course, would only apply to undue prescribing when the doctor had a considerable financial interest, e.g. as a director of a company. It does not refer to the doctor who holds a few shares in some drug company.

Profiting at the expense of his colleagues

Canvassing. Although it is perfectly normal in commerce for a business man to send circulars to potential clients indicating in laudatory terms the value and scope of his services, such behaviour on the part of a doctor would constitute infamous conduct. Neither should he attempt to attract another doctor's patients to his own practice by word of mouth, or any other means.

It is, of course, permissible to inform patients on the doctor's own list of a change in the doctor's address or telephone number, but such notification should be confined to a simple statement of the alteration, and should be sent in an envelope to ensure that it is only seen by the person for whom it was intended.

Advertising. The blatant forms of advertising such as advertisements or articles on the lay press drawing attention to a doctor's abilities, or large and elaborate signs at his surgery are obvious and fortunately rare.

More difficult problems arise in the fields of broadcasting and the writing of books and articles intended to be read by the general public, and in lecturing to lay audiences. To remain anonymous is usually the best safeguard against accusations of advertising, at the same time ensuring that nothing said or written by the doctor could be interpreted as being directed towards his own personal advantage. The doctor must also exercise care with regard to advertising if he works for any of the modern forms of private 'health clinic'.

Deprecation of other doctors. Whether criticism of another doctor is justified or not, it should never be made in the presence of patients or members of the public. If a doctor feels that one of his colleagues is deserving of censure, his correct course is to inform the GMC.

Ethical advice

Under the Medical Act 1983 the GMC has the duty to provide advice to the profession on standards of professional conduct and medical ethics. At the present time it does this through the Standards Committee by including a section of such advice in the pamphlet *Professional Conduct and Discipline: Fitness to Practice*, which it issues at regular intervals, and also in its annual report. This provides detailed guidance on such matters as advertising, for instance with regard to articles or books, or broadcasting or television appearances, and should be consulted in the original for further detail. Some of the most recent advice has been in connection with doctors' attitudes to persons suffering from AIDS.

Disciplinary procedure

Notifications of convictions of doctors and complaints of their misconduct are received by the Registrar and submitted by him to the President, or another member of the Council (the Preliminary Screener for conduct cases). The Council's solicitor may be asked to make further enquiries at this stage. If then the matter is considered trivial it may be dismissed. Otherwise the doctor is informed if an allegation of misconduct has been made against him, of the nature of the allegation and invited to submit a written explanation. This explanation, and other evidence in the case is then referred to the Preliminary Proceedings Committee.

Preliminary Proceedings Committee

This consists of 11 members, elected annually. It is advised on legal matters by a Legal Assessor. Its function is to make preliminary enquiry into the case, to judge whether it merits further investigation.

Allegations of professional misconduct must be supported by a statutory declaration, unless the allegation is made by a person acting in a public capacity, e.g. an officer of a government department or a local authority.

After considering the case the Committee may take no further action. In cases where the infringement of professional conduct does not appear to be too serious the Committee will send the doctor a warning letter. If the matter appears more serious they will usually refer the case to the Professional Conduct Committee, but in the event of apparent impairment of the doctor's physical or mental condition they may refer it to the Health Committee.

The Preliminary Proceedings Committee may order interim suspension of the doctor's registration, or his conditional registration, for a period of up to 2 months, until the case can be dealt with by the Professional Conduct or the Health Committee; if it does the doctor must first be given the opportunity of appearing before the Committee, and may be legally represented.

Professional Conduct Committee

This Committee consists of 20 members, of whom two are lay members. Only ten members take part in any one case. The Committee is advised on legal matters by a Legal Assessor.

The procedure of the Committee is similar to that of a Court of Law. The doctor is entitled to be legally represented. Witnesses may be subpoenaed to attend and give evidence on oath.

If the Committee is considering the conviction of a doctor (in a Court of Law), it is bound to accept the fact of conviction as proof that the doctor was guilty of the offence charged. Similarly the finding in a matrimonial court of adultery by a doctor is proof of the fact. The Committee's purpose in such a case is to decide whether the nature of the offence or conduct merits erasure of the doctor's name from the Register. In cases of alleged infamous conduct evidence may be called before the Committee from either side to determine the truth of the allegation.

Having considered the facts the Committee may receive evidence in mitigation from the accused doctor. It then has to decide whether the facts justify any punitive action against the doctor. If so, the committee has several possible courses of action. It may direct that the doctor's name be erased from the Register. It can direct that his registration be suspended for up to 12 months. His registration can be made conditional upon his complying with certain restrictions imposed by the Committee, for up to 3 years. A form of probation exists whereby the Committee postpones its decision for a stated interval, e.g. 6 months, at which time the facts are reconsidered and evidence of the doctor's behaviour during the interval is produced, before a final decision is made. This course of action may be deemed appropriate in some cases of alcoholism or drug addiction. Finally, the Committee may admonish the doctor and conclude the case.

If the judgement is postponed, or the doctor's registration made conditional, he remains on the Register and may practise as a doctor. In the case of suspension, as with erasure of registration he may no longer practise as a registered medical practitioner.

Under new legislation a practitioner from another member state of the EEC can be banned from registration, or erased from the Register if there is a disqualifying decision against him in the state from which he originates.

Appeals

The doctor whose registration is to be erased, or suspended or made conditional may appeal to the Judicial Committee of the Privy Council against the decision. Such an appeal must be lodged within 28 days of the decision. But the Professional Conduct Committee may order the doctor's registration to be suspended forthwith in extreme cases, where it is satisfied that such action is justified in the interests of the public, or the doctor himself.

Restoration after erasure

A doctor whose name has been erased from the Register after disciplinary proceedings may apply to have his name restored at any time after 10

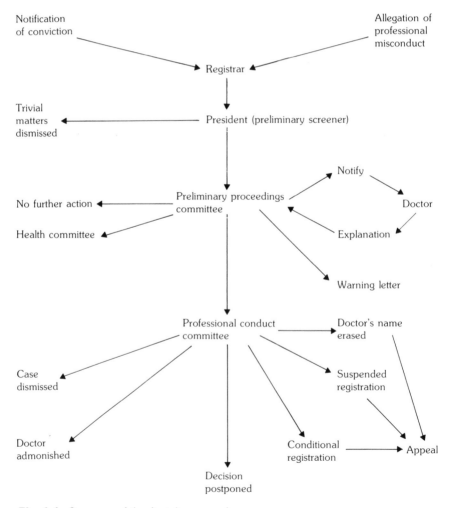

Fig. 1.1. Summary of the discipline procedure.

months from the date of erasure, and if unsuccessful at 10 monthly intervals thereafter. Such restoration is not unusual if evidence of satisfactory behaviour subsequent to erasure is available, and the original offence was not too grave.

Complaints under the NHS

In addition to the GMC, procedures exist whereby a doctor working in the NHS may be called upon to answer a complaint, either by the Family Practitioner Committee, if he is a general practitioner; or by the district Administrator or Health Service Commissioner if he works in a hospital. The enquiries may result in a reprimand or the withholding of some remuneration from the doctor. Enquiries may also be made by the Health Services Committee Ombudsman.

Chapter 2
Certification of Death and
Disposal Procedure

The legal procedure, following a death, may be summarised as follows:

1   The cause of death must be ascertained and certified by a death certificate or determined by a Coroner's investigation.

2   Details of the death and of the deceased are recorded by the Registrar of Births and Deaths.

3   The body must be disposed of, by any lawful means. This may be done by earth burial, sea burial or by cremation.

Notification of the cause of death

Death certificate

Regulations for the issue of death certificates have existed since 1874. The object of the certificates is to prevent the concealment of crime, and to obtain information, for statistical purposes, of causes of death in the population.

When may a doctor issue a death certificate?

1   If he is a registered medical practitioner.

2   If he attended the deceased during the last illness. In practice this usually means where the doctor attended within 14 days of the death. In some cases when the doctor was attending the deceased regularly *and had seen the body after death*, the certificate may be accepted even though the last attendance was more than 14 days before death. A practitioner who sees the deceased for the first time after death, such as a locum, or a partner of the usual medical attendant, is not entitled to issue a certificate.

3   If he knows the cause of death. According to the law, if the two previous criteria are satisfied the doctor must always issue a certificate, even if the cause is unknown or obviously unnatural. The Registrar would then notify the Coroner. However, the usual practice in such cases is for the doctor to notify the Coroner himself, and withhold the certificate.

The form of the certificate

The certificate must be in the form prescribed by the Registrar General (Fig. 2.2) and books of such certificates, together with the franked envelopes for their dispatch, can be obtained from the local Registrar of Births and Deaths.

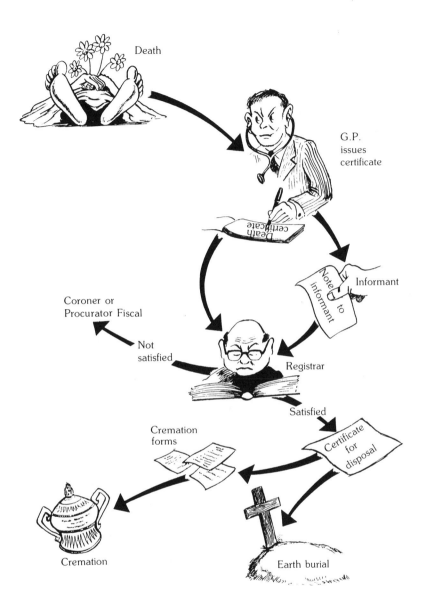

Fig. 2.1. Disposal procedure by certification.

Note

1 The doctor is not at present obliged to see the body after death before issuing the certificate. It is advisable to do so, however, in case the death has resulted from some injury sustained since the doctor last visited, or lest death has not in fact occurred.

Side 1

MEDA 14   000000

Register to enter
No. of Death Entry.

BIRTHS AND DEATHS REGISTRATION ACT 1953

(Form prescribed by the Registration of Births, Deaths and Marriages (Amendment) Regulations 1985)

MEDICAL CERTIFICATE OF CAUSE OF DEATH

For use only by a Registered Medical Practitioner WHO HAS BEEN IN ATTENDANCE during the deceased's last illness, and to be delivered by him forthwith to the Registrar of Births and Deaths.

Name of deceased ....

Date of death as stated to me .... day of .... 19 ....

Place of death .... day of ....

Last seen alive by me .... day of ....   Age as stated to me ....

1 The certified cause of death takes account of information obtained from post-mortem.

2 Information from post-mortem may be available later.

3 Post-mortem not being held.

4 I have reported this death to the Coroner for further action.

[See overleaf]

a Seen after death by me.

b Seen after death by another medical practitioner.

c Not seen after death by me.

d Not seen after death by a medical practitioner.

Please ring appropriate digit(s) and letter

CAUSE OF DEATH

The condition thought to be the Underlying Cause of Death should appear in the lowest completed line of Part I

These particulars not to be entered in death register

Approximate interval between onset and death

I(a) Disease or condition directly leading to death†   ....

(b) Other disease or condition, if any, leading to I(a)   ....

(c) Other disease or condition, if any, leading to I(b)   ....

II Other significant conditions CONTRIBUTING TO THE DEATH but not related to the disease or condition causing it   ....

The death might have been due to or contributed to by the employment followed at some time by the deceased

Please tick where applicable ☐

† *This does not mean the mode of dying, such as heart failure, asphyxia, asthenia, etc. it means the disease, injury, or complication which caused death*

I hereby certify that I was in medical attendance during the above named deceased's last illness, and that the particulars and cause of death above written are true to the best of my knowledge and belief.

Signature .... Qualifications as registered by General Medical Council }

Residence .... Date ....

For deaths in hospital: Please give the name of the consultant responsible for the above-named as a patient ....

MEDA 14   000000

(Form prescribed by the Registration of Births, Deaths and Marriages Regulations 1968)

NOTICE TO INFORMANT

I hereby give notice that I have this day signed a medical certificate of cause of death of

....

Signature ....

Date ....

This notice is to be delivered by the informant to the registrar of births and deaths for the sub-district in which the death occurred.

The certifying medical practitioner must give this notice to the person who is qualified and liable to act as informant for the registration of death (see list overleaf).

DUTIES OF INFORMANT

Failure to deliver this notice to the registrar renders the informant liable to prosecution. The death cannot be registered until the medical certificate has reached the registrar.

When the death is registered the informant must be prepared to give to the registrar the following particulars relating to the deceased

1 The date and place of death

2 The full name and surname (and the maiden surname if the deceased was a woman who had married)

3 The date and place of birth

4 The occupation (and if the deceased was a married woman or a widow the name and occupation of her husband)

5 The usual address.

6 Whether the deceased was in receipt of a pension or allowance from public funds.

7 If the deceased was married, the date of birth of the surviving widow or widower.

THE DECEASED'S MEDICAL CARD SHOULD BE DELIVERED TO THE REGISTRAR

Side 2

Complete where applicable

A

I have reported this death to the Coroner for further action.

Initials of certifying medical practitioner

The Coroner needs to consider all cases where:

The death might have been due to or contributed to by a violent or unnatural cause (including an accident);

or the cause of death cannot be identified;

or the death might have been due to or contributed to by drugs, medicine, abortion or poison.

B

I may be in a position later to give, on application by the Registrar General, additional information as to the cause of death for the purpose of more precise statistical classification

Initials of certifying medical practitioner

or there is reason to believe that the death occurred during an operation or under or prior to complete recovery from an anaesthetic or arising subsequently out of an incident during an operation or an anaesthetic;

or the death might have been due to or contributed to by the employment followed at some time by the deceased

PERSONS QUALIFIED AND LIABLE TO ACT AS INFORMANTS

The following persons are designated by the Births and Deaths Registration Act 1953 as qualified to give information concerning a death—

DEATHS IN HOUSES AND PUBLIC INSTITUTIONS

(1) A relative of the deceased, present at the death

(2) A relative of the deceased, in attendance during the last illness.

(3) A relative of the deceased, residing or being in the sub-district where the death occurred

(4) A person present at the death

(5) The occupier* if he knew of the happening of the death

(6) Any inmate if he knew of the happening of the death

(7) The person causing the disposal of the body.

DEATHS NOT IN HOUSES OR DEAD BODIES FOUND

(1) Any relative of the deceased having knowledge of any of the particulars required to be registered.

(2) Any person present at the death

(3) Any person who found the body.

(4) Any person in charge of the body.

(5) The person causing the disposal of the body.

*"Occupier" in relation to a public institution includes the governor, keeper, master, matron, superintendent or other chief resident officer

LIST OF SOME OF THE CATEGORIES OF DEATH WHICH MAY BE OF INDUSTRIAL ORIGIN

MALIGNANT DISEASES	Causes include	INFECTIOUS DISEASES	Causes include
(a) Skin	– radiation and sunlight – pitch or tar – mineral oils	(a) Anthrax	imported hides, bonemeal, hide or fur
(b) Nasal	– wood or leather work – nickel	(b) Brucellosis	farming or veterinary
(c) Lung	– asbestos – nickel – radiation	(c) Tuberculosis	contact at work
(d) Pleura	– asbestos	(d) Leptospirosis	farming, sewer or underground workers
(e) Urinary Tract	– benzidine – dyestuff – chemicals in rubbers	(e) Tetanus	farming or gardening
(f) Liver	– PVC manufacture	(f) Rabies	animal handling
(g) Bone	– radiation	(g) Viral hepatitis	contact at work
(h) Lymphatics and haematopoietic	– radiation – benzene	BRONCHIAL ASTHMA AND PNEUMONITIS	
POISONING		(a) Occupational asthma	sensitising agent at work
(a) Metals	e.g. arsenic, cadmium, lead	(b) Allergic Alveolitis	farming
(b) Chemicals	e.g. chlorine, benzene	PNEUMOCONIOSIS	mining and quarrying, pottery, asbestos
(c) Solvents	e.g. trichlorethylene		

NOTE:—The Practitioner, on signing the certificate, should complete, sign and date the Notice to the Informant, which should be detached and handed to the Informant. The Practitioner should then, without delay, deliver the certificate itself to the Registrar of Births and Deaths for the sub-district in which the death occurred. Envelopes for enclosing the certificates are supplied by the Registrar

Fig. 2.2. Medical certificate of cause of death (reproduced courtesy of HMSO).

2   When stating the cause of death, precise terms of the responsible morbid conditions, e.g. cerebral haemorrhage or coronary thrombosis, should be used. Vague terms, such as asphyxia or heart failure, are not acceptable. The book of certificates contains a list of undesirable terms. If the terminal event is a consequence of pre-existing diseases, these must be recorded in the correct sequence, e.g.

	Ia Cerebral haemorrhage
due to	Ib Hypertension
due to	Ic Chronic nephritis

Any other condition independently contributing to death, but not forming part of the sequence, should be noted in Part II, e.g.

II Chronic bronchitis

Examples of correct certification are given in the book of certificates for the guidance of doctors. Newly qualified doctors often find difficulty in deciding the correct way to fill up this part of the certificate. This may be due to failure to identify the main underlying disease or condition originally starting the process leading to death, such as a carcinoma of the bladder which may eventually cause death from a bewildering variety of conditions such as biochemical disturbances and pulmonary complications. Secondly, the doctor may fail to appreciate the relevance of an unnatural factor in the death, even when the relationship in time is remote, as with the development of a mesothelioma many years after exposure to asbestos.

3   If any of the conditions listed in Parts I and II may have an unnatural cause, the Registrar will refer the case of the Coroner. Therefore ambiguous terms such as 'gangrene' or 'cirrhosis' should be qualified by an indication of the cause, e.g. cardiac cirrhosis or alcoholic cirrhosis.

4   The spaces A and B on the reverse of the form are likely to be rarely used. The doctor should initial A when he has both notified the Coroner and also issued a death certificate, a practice which is strictly correct but hardly ever followed. Space B should be initialled if he is awaiting the results of some laboratory investigation, e.g. histology, which may provide additional information of value for statistical purposes.

5   The qualifications which the doctor appends must only be those entered in the Medical Register.

6   Certification is to the best of the doctor's belief and knowledge. Subsequent demonstration that his diagnosis was incorrect does not make him guilty of an offence. Nevertheless, he must use the utmost care in completing the certificate.

7   On completion of the certificate the doctor retains a counterfoil, sends the certificate to the Registrar, and detaches and hands the Notice to Informant (see below) to the appropriate person.

8   The certificate is a statutory document, i.e. required under the Births and Deaths Registration Act. No fee may be charged by the doctor, but he may be prosecuted for failure to issue a certificate if he is eligible to do so.

The report of a Home Office committee, the 'Brodrick Report' on death certification and Coroners, recommends many alterations to the procedure for disposal, including the use of a much more comprehensive certificate of cause of death, and the abolition of the cremation forms. There is, as yet, no sign of implementation of its recommendations except as regards a few aspects of Coroner's practice.

The informant

This is the person whose duty it is to register the death. Usually he is a relative of the deceased, but the back of the Notice to Informant bears a list of people who may be required to act if no relative is available, e.g. the person causing the disposal of the body. The informant must take the Notice to the Registrar, and register the death within 5 days.

Still-Birth Certificate

By law any registered medical practitioner or certified midwife who was present at a still-birth, or examines the body of a still-born child must give to the person qualified to act as informant for the purpose of registration, a certificate of still-birth, in the prescribed form (Fig. 2.3).

If the informant cannot for any reason obtain such a certificate he may make a statutory declaration of still-birth to the Registrar and explain why the certificate is not available. This anachronism is unlikely to be used nowadays.

The definition of a still-born child is a child which has been born after the twenty-eighth week of pregnancy and which did not, after having been completely expelled from its mother, breathe or show any other sign of life. Signs of life, in addition to breathing, are movement, heart beat, or pulsation of the umbilical cord.

As in the case of death certificates, still-birth certificates are obtainable from the Registrar of Births and Deaths in book form.

Note

1   In stating the cause of death, indefinite terms must be avoided. (Examples are given in the book of certificates.) The nomenclature of the International Classification of Causes of Still-Birth should be used.

2   If the doctor was not present at the birth, he should be very cautious before forming an opinion of still-birth on external examination of the body,

MEDICAL CERTIFICATE OF STILL-BIRTH

(Births and Deaths Registration Act 1953, S 11 (1), as amended by the Population (Statistics) Act 1960)
(Form prescribed by the Registration of Births, Deaths and Marriages Regulations 1968)

SB   354073

To be given only in respect of a child which has issued forth from its mother after the 28th week of pregnancy and which did not at any time after being completely expelled from its mother breathe or show any other signs of life.

| Registered at |
| Entry No. |

*I was present at the still-birth of a $\frac{*male}{*female}$ child born

*I have examined the body of a $\frac{*male}{*female}$ child which I am informed and believe was born

on the ....day of.................................19.......to.....................................

(NAME OF MOTHER)

at ....

(PLACE OF BIRTH)

I hereby certify that (i) the child was not born alive, and
(ii) to the best of my knowledge and belief the cause of death and the estimated duration of pregnancy of the mother were as stated below.

CAUSE OF DEATH	Estimated duration of pregnancy
DIRECT CAUSE State foetal or maternal condition directly $\left.\right\}$ (a) causing death.	weeks
ANTECEDENT CAUSES State foetal and/or maternal conditions, if (b) any, giving rise to the above cause, due to stating the underlying cause last. (c)	**Weight of foetus (if known)**
OTHER SIGNIFICANT CONDITIONS of foetus or mother which may have contributed to but, in so far as is known, were not related to direct cause of death.	lbs. oz.

†{ 1 The certified cause of death has been confirmed by post-mortem.
2 Post-mortem information may be available later.
3 Post-mortem not being held.

Signature ....   Date ....

Qualification as registered by General Medical Council, $\left.\right\}$ or Registered No. as Certified Midwife.

Residence ....

*Strike out the words which do not apply.
†Ring appropriate digit.

THIS IS NOT AN AUTHORITY FOR BURIAL OR CREMATION

[SEE OVER

Fig. 2.3. Medical certificate of still-birth (reproduced courtesy of HMSO).

unless some obvious congenital malformation incompatible with life, or maceration of the body, is present. Any uncertainty is best resolved by reference to the Coroner.

3   There is a counterfoil to the certificate, but no Notice to Informant. The doctor hands the completed certificate to the informant instead of sending it to the Registrar.

4   The informant may be: the mother; the father of a legitimate child; a person present at the birth; the occupier of the house in which the birth occurred.

5   The still-birth must be registered within 42 days and the birth must be notified to the Medical Officer of Health.

Notification of a death to the Coroner or Procurator Fiscal

The doctor has no statutory duty to notify any death to the Coroner. He complies with the law if he issues a death certificate, even though the death

Side 2

NOTE TO INFORMANT

Under Section 11(1) of the Births and Deaths Registration Act 1953, this certificate must be delivered to the Registrar of Births and Deaths by the person attending to give information of the particulars required to be registered concerning the still-birth. The persons qualified and liable to give such information include:

(1) the mother;

(2) the father (of a legitimate child only);

(3) the occupier of the house in which to the knowledge of that occupier the still-birth occurred;*

(4) a person present at the still-birth;

(5) the person in charge of the still-born child.

The still-birth is required to be registered within 42 days of its occurrence.

*Occupier in relation to a public institution includes the governor, keeper, master, matron, superintendent, or other chief resident officer.

is due to an unnatural cause, and leaves the Registrar to inform the Coroner. There is, however, a duty in Common Law for every person 'about a body' to notify the Coroner of circumstances likely to require the holding of an inquest, but this duty is not enforceable. The generally accepted practice is for the doctor personally to notify the Coroner of a death and not to issue a death certificate, avoiding thereby much inconvenience and waste of time (Fig 2.4).

There is no official list to guide the doctor in deciding when to refer a death to the Coroner. A simple rule is to refer all deaths known to be due to unnatural causes, or when the cause is unknown. Examples of the type of death which *should* be referred are as follows:

1 Deaths from violence—accidental, suicidal or homicidal. This applies whether death results immediately and directly from the injury, or is indirectly related, after a lapse of weeks, months or even years.

2 Deaths following abortion.

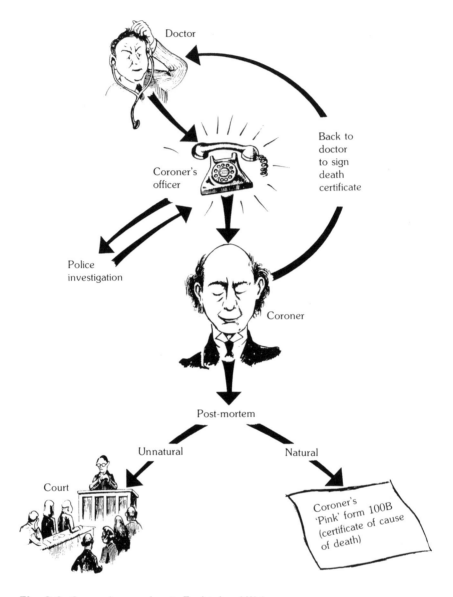

Fig. 2.4. Coroner's procedure in England and Wales.

3 Deaths from privation or neglect—including self-neglect.
4 Deaths from poison and alcoholism.
5 Deaths during surgical operation or anaesthesia.
6 Deaths from industrial disease.
7 Deaths of persons in receipt of war pensions.
8 Deaths from unknown causes.
(For the procedure of Coroner's Investigations see Chapter 10.)

Registration of death

The informant must attend the Registrar, to give details of the deceased to be entered on the Register, and to hand to the Registrar certain documents, such as the medical card and any papers relating to pensions received by the deceased from National Funds, e.g. war pensions. The Registrar will record the cause of death as given on the death certificate. He has a statutory obligation to inform the Coroner of deaths in certain circumstances, as when the cause of death appears to have been unnatural, or if the deceased had not been attended by a medical practitioner during his last illness. Death certificates containing ambiguous terms which might indicate an unnatural cause, e.g. cirrhosis of the liver, will undoubtedly cause the death to be referred to the Coroner.

If the Registrar is satisfied that there is no need for further enquiry into the death, he will authorise disposal of the body by issuing a certificate for Disposal after Registry. Disposal of a body without authorisation from the Registrar or the Coroner is illegal.

Procedure in Scotland, Eire and Northern Ireland

In Scotland a death certificate may be issued by any doctor who knows the cause of death, even if he was not in attendance during the last illness. Deaths from unnatural or unknown cause are referred to the Procurator Fiscal, who takes the place of the English Coroner. The death certificate is different in form (Figs. 2.5, 2.6), and has no notice to informant. It must be delivered to the Registrar within 7 days of the death. It is not necessary to deliver the certificate immediately, or 'forthwith' as in England, and in fact a burial may take place before the registration is effected, provided the Registrar is informed beforehand.

In Eire, under the provisions of the Coroner's Act of 1962, a medical practitioner must notify the Coroner of the death of a patient whom he has not attended during the preceding month, or whom he knows to have died of one of a list of specified conditions.

In Northern Ireland there is no provision for an Informant, and the length of the 'last illness', during which time before death the doctor should have seen the deceased, if he is to issue a certificate is 28 days, not 14 as in England.

Disposal of the body

Burial

The Registrar's certificate for disposal is delivered to the person arranging the funeral, e.g. the undertaker. After burial a notification of disposal is sent by the undertaker to the Registrar.

The duty to arrange for disposal of the body is usually that of the

Side 1

MEDICAL CERTIFICATE OF CAUSE OF DEATH   FORM 11

This certificate is intended for the use of the Registrar of Births, Deaths and Marriages, and all persons are warned against accepting or using this certificate for any other purpose. See back of this form for notes about registration of a death.

To the Registrar of Births, Deaths and Marriages

I hereby certify that

Counterfoil

Name of deceased

Registrar to enter:
Dist No
Year
Entry No

died at   hours   on   19
                time   date

at
        place of death

Date of Death

and that to the best of my knowledge and belief, the cause of death and duration of disease were as stated below

Place of Death

CAUSE OF DEATH   (Please print clearly)

Disease or condition directly leading to death*

a   due to (or as a consequence of)

Antecedent causes
Morbid conditions, if any, giving rise to the above cause, the underlying condition to be stated last

b   due to (or as a consequence of)

c   due to (or as a consequence of)

Other significant conditions
contributing to the death, but not related to the disease or condition causing it

Cause of Death

I a

b

c

II

Not to be entered in register

Approximate interval between onset and death

years   months   days

*This does not mean the mode of dying such as heart failure, asthenia, etc. It means the disease, injury or complication which caused death

Please ring appropriate letter and appropriate figure:—
Certified cause takes account of post-mortem information   A
Information from post-mortem may be available later   B
Post-mortem not proposed   C

Seen after death by me   1
Seen after death by another medical practitioner but not by me 2
Not seen after death by a medical practitioner   3

If deceased was a married woman and death occurred during pregnancy, or within six weeks thereafter, write Yes

Signature

Date   19

Name in BLOCK CAPITALS

Registered medical qualifications

Address

P—M ring letter   A   B   C

Seen after death   1   2   3
ring figure

Pregnancy

Date of Certification

D2(R)
983

Side 2

NOTES ABOUT REGISTRATION OF A DEATH

A death may be registered either in the registration district where it takes place (the district of its occurrence) or in such other registration district in Scotland where the deceased person had his usual residence immediately before his death.

Usual residence for this purpose means the deceased person's permanent home and not an address (e.g. a holiday address) at which he may have been staying temporarily at the time of his death.

Persons required to give information for the registration of a death are:

a   any relative of the deceased;

b   any person present at the death;

c   the deceased's executor or other legal representative;

d   the occupier, at the time of death, of the premises where the death took place;

e   if there is no such person as aforesaid, any other person having knowledge of the particulars to be registered.

N.B. The word 'occupier' includes the governor, keeper, matron, superintendent or other person in charge of a prison, hospital or other institution, and, in relation to a house, includes any person residing therein.

Fig. 2.5. Scottish medical certificate of cause of death (reproduced courtesy of the Registrar General for Scotland).

Side 1

Medical Certificate of Cause of Death   Form 11   Specimen

D2(R)

Registration of Births, Deaths and Marriages (Scotland) Act 1965, section 24

This is a specimen copy of the form "Medical Certificate of Cause of Death" and of the notes and examples which are included in the book of forms. The book of forms issued to doctors has a blue cover and contains twenty forms and a page showing the notes and examples which follow.

Note to certifier

General

1. Many important advances in medicine have been initiated as a result of studies based on data from medical certification of cause of death. As diagnostic methods become more precise and as methods of analysis become more efficient it is likely that such studies will become more valuable. The most important stage in these studies is the recording of the basic information and it is therefore important that medical certification of cause of death should be carried out with care and that the form of certification should be consistent and clear.

The International Certificate

2. The adoption in Scotland of the international form of medical certificate of cause of death has been in response to representations made by the Scottish medical profession. This form is considered to have the advantages that it permits international comparability, that its sequence is a logical one for the certifying practitioner and that it permits a more informative analysis of the collected data deriving from such certificates.

3. The international form of medical certificate of cause of death is divided into two parts. The first (Part I) describes the sequence of morbid conditions directly leading to death; the second (Part II) describes other morbid conditions which may have contributed to the death, but which were not involved in the fatal sequence.

4. In using Part I to describe the fatal sequence, the condition directly leading to death is recorded first at II(a). This condition may be a complication or consequence of preexisting or underlying conditions or may itself represent the underlying cause of death. If the latter is the case then no more need be entered in Part I. But if the immediate condition causing death is a complication or consequence of an underlying condition, this underlying condition should be recorded next. If this in turn arose from a further underlying condition then this latter should in turn be recorded next so that the **underlying cause of death** or the condition initiating the fatal sequence is recorded last.

5. If other conditions contributed to the fatal outcome but were not directly involved in the fatal sequence, they should be recorded in Part II.

6. It is recognised that there are cases where it may be difficult to decide whether a condition present at death should be regarded as part of the fatal sequence leading to death or whether it should be regarded as a contributory condition appropriately assignable to Part II. It should be noted that the conditions entered in Part I should represent a distinct sequence so that each condition entered may be regarded as being a direct consequence of the condition entered below it. Where a condition present at death does not seem to fit into such a sequence it should be recorded in Part II. Examples are given which illustrate the principles involved.

Maternal conditions as causes of death in the newborn

7. In general, disease conditions recorded on a death certificate will be conditions from which the deceased suffered. However, in certifying the cause of death of a newborn infant the practitioner may wish to record underlying conditions in the mother of the deceased infant. This may be done, although it is expected that maternal conditions will usually be regarded as a cause of infant death only in the first 28 days of life. Where maternal conditions are recorded, they should be distinguished as "maternal", as in the example.

Terminology

8. The basic point is that the cause of death to be recorded on a medical certificate should reflect the considered opinion of the certifying practitioner.

9. The causes a practitioner gives will for tabulation purposes be assigned by the office of the Registrar General to the appropriate rubrics of the International Classification of Diseases, Injuries or Causes of Death. It is not desired, however, that practitioners should necessarily adopt the terms used in this classification. If the classification does not conveniently accommodate the diagnostic terms prevalent in contemporary medicine, it is the classification which requires

revision, rather than the prevailing terminology. The classification is subject to decennial revision by the World Health Organisation and member nations are represented on the revision committees.

10. It is hoped that the quality of the information recorded will be as high as that considered appropriate in records kept in clinical practice. Certifying practitioners are asked therefore to be as specific as they are able; for example they should specify the primary site of tumours, and they should distinguish where appropriate between acute and chronic or other varieties of a disease.

11. The causes recorded on medical certificates of cause of death are analysed and tabulated so as to permit the identification of areas of further enquiry likely to lead to advances in preventive or curative medicine. The usefulness of these analyses depends directly on the care with which causes are identified and recorded and in order to ensure that no cause is assigned to the classification inaccurately, practitioners are asked not to contract or symbolise causes of death.

Further information on cause of death

12. The office of the Registrar General may communicate with the certifying practitioner either if further classification or amplification of the certified cause seems desirable or if the practitioner has indicated on the certificate that further information may be available from post-mortem examination.

13. In a case where a practitioner has not ringed letter "B" on the certificate to indicate that post-mortem information may be available later, but for any reason subsequently decides that the certified cause requires to be amplified or amended, it would be appreciated if he intimated the fact to the Registrar General, Vital Statistics Branch, Ladywell House, Ladywell Road, Edinburgh, EH12 7TF.

As the particulars of the cause of death, and the name of the certifying doctor as signed by him, are transcribed by the Registrar into his register of Deaths, it would be extremely helpful if the doctor would repeat, in block capitals, his signature appearing on the certificate.

Side 2

EXAMPLES OF THE USE OF THE INTERNATIONAL MEDICAL CERTIFICATE OF CAUSE OF DEATH

1. A patient with chronic peptic ulceration dies of peritonitis a few days after an operation for perforation of a duodenal ulcer.

  I. (a) Peritonitis.
      (b) Perforation of duodenal ulcer (operation).
      (c) Peptic ulcer of the duodenum.
  II. –

2. A patient with acute intestinal obstruction from a carcinoma of the rectum and severe chronic bronchitis with emphysema dies during an operation to relieve the intestinal obstruction.

  I. (a) Intestinal obstruction - died during operation (anaesthetic—thiopentone, halothane).
      (b) Carcinoma of the rectum.
  II. Chronic bronchitis and emphysema.

NOTE– The sequence of events leading to death was initiated by the carcinoma of the rectum. Although it may be thought that the patient would have survived the operation had it not been for his bronchitis and emphysema, these conditions would not be regarded as part of the fatal sequence.

3. A patient suffering from a residual hemiparesis following a cerebral thrombosis several years ago falls at home and sustains a fracture of the neck of the femur. During immobilisation following this injury the patient develops hypostatic pneumonia from which he dies.

  I. (a) Hypostatic pneumonia.
      (b) Immobilisation.
      (c) Fracture of the neck of the femur (accidental fall at home).
  II. Hemiparesis - old cerebral thrombosis.

4. A patient with a long standing severe hypertension with compensated congestive cardiac failure and history of cardiac asthma dies following a short illness characterised by sudden onset of hemiplegia and loss of speech.

  I. (a) Cerebral vascular accident.
      (b) –
      (c) –
  II. Hypertension.
        Hypertensive heart disease.

5. A patient is accidentally run over by a 'bus and sustains extensive abdominal injuries necessitating surgical correction involving hospitalisation on several occasions over a period of several months. During recovery from one such operation the patient dies suddenly of a pulmonary embolus.

  I. (a) Pulmonary embolus following operation.
      (b) Gross trauma to abdominal organs (accident - run over by 'bus).
  II. –

6. An infant dies shortly after birth as a result of intra-natal anoxia due to maternal toxaemia of pregnancy. The infant was prematurely born.

  I. (a) Intra-natal anoxia.
      (b) Maternal toxaemia of pregnancy.
  II. Prematurity.

THE REGISTRATION OF BIRTHS, DEATHS AND MARRIAGES (SCOTLAND) ACT 1965

SECTION 24 – (1) For the purpose of enabling information to be given, in pursuance of the last foregoing section, of the cause of death of any person, any registered medical practitioner who was in attendance on the deceased during his last illness shall, within seven days, or such other period, not being less than two days, as may be prescribed, after the death of the person, transmit to any person who is a qualified informant in relation to the death, or to the registrar, a certificate in the prescribed form signed by the medical practitioner stating to the best of his knowledge and belief the cause of death.

Different forms of certificate may be prescribed in respect of persons of different ages, and in the case of the death of a child under one year of age such forms may provide for the giving of particulars of the condition of the mother before the death of the child.

(2) If there was no registered medical practitioner in attendance on the deceased during his last illness, or if any registered medical practitioner, having been in attendance as aforesaid, is unable to provide a certificate such as is required by the last foregoing subsection, such a certificate may be signed by any medical practitioner who is able to do so, and may be transmitted by him to any person who is a qualified informant in relation to the death, or to the registrar.

Note: It is very desirable that the medical certificate should be issued as soon as possible after the occurrence of the death to which it relates. Books of medical certificate forms (Form II) may be obtained by registered medical practitioners from the Registrar of Births, Deaths and Marriages of the registration district in which they practise.

Fig. 2.6. Scottish medical certificate of cause of death — notes and examples (reproduced courtesy of the Registrar General for Scotland).

executor, or the next of kin of an intestate. The local authority must act if no-one is available, e.g. in the case of a person without relatives. A Death Grant is no longer provided to cover the cost of disposal. Instead, help can be obtained from the Social Fund.

Cremation

First a medical certificate of cause of death must be issued, the death must be registered and the Registrar's certificate for disposal must be obtained. In addition, application must be made to the cremation authorities for cremation of the body, by submission of several different forms. The more stringent regulations applied to this method of disposal are designed to ensure that evidence of crime is not destroyed, and that cremation is not carried out against the wishes of the deceased or a relative.

Form A. The application for cremation, submitted by the person having the duty to dispose of the body. Any objections to cremation known to have been made by the deceased or any relative and any reason to believe that death was due to violence, poison, or neglect, or that a further examination of the body is necessary must be stated. The form is countersigned by a person in authority, e.g. an MP, or a police officer, who knows the applicant.

Form B. A medical certificate given by the doctor who issued the death certificate. Details are required of the mode of dying as well as the cause of death, and the doctor must have examined the body after death. He must disclose any relationship he had to the deceased, and any pecuniary interest which he may have in the death.

Form C. A confirmatory medical certificate given by a practitioner of at least 5 years' registration. He must not be related to the deceased or to the doctor issuing form B. He also must examine the body after death, and see and question the doctor giving form B.

Both doctors must state that they have no reason to believe that the death was due to any unnatural cause, or that any further examination of the body is necessary. Under new regulations, if a post-mortem examination has been carried out in a hospital by a pathologist of at least 5 years' registration, and the results are notified to the doctor completing Form B, these details may be inserted into Form B and then there is no need for Form C to be completed.

Form F. The authority to cremate. It is issued by the medical referee of the cremation authority (who may also be the local community physician) after scrutiny of the previous forms, when he is satisfied that all requirements of the cremation regulations have been fulfilled.

After cremation a certificate of disposal is sent to the Registrar, as in the case of burial.

Special forms

Form D. A certificate of cause of death issued after a post-mortem examination, ordered or performed by the medical referee when he has considered further investigation of the cause of death to be necessary. It replaces forms B and C, but is rarely used in England and Wales.

Form E. The Coroner's certificate of cause of death, or the appropriate form from the Procurator Fiscal issued after a post-mortem examination has been made at his direction, or an inquest has been held. It replaces the medical certificates on forms B and C, but not form F. It is not the authority to cremate.

Disposal in special circumstances

Anatomical dissection

The procedure to be followed, as laid down by the Anatomy Acts, is complicated. If a patient expresses a wish that his body should be used for dissection, the doctor should advise him to contact the local teacher of anatomy, e.g. the Professor of Anatomy in a medical school who will supply the relevant forms, and explain the procedure. If the patient merely indicates his wishes in his will, and no arrangements are made before his death, difficulties are likely to arise.

Disposal of parts of a body—Human Tissue Act 1961

This Act makes lawful the removal of tissues of a deceased person for therapeutic purposes and for medical education and research. It replaced the Corneal Grafting Act of 1952. It also permits the performance of post-mortem examinations to establish or confirm the cause of death, provided that the death is not one which should be notified to the Coroner or Procurator Fiscal.

Removal of tissues

Tissues may be removed if the deceased requested this in writing at any time, or orally during his or her last illness in the presence of two or more witnesses.

If no such request had been made, the person lawfully in possession of the body, i.e. the hospital management committee or board of governors, may authorise the removal of tissues provided that there is no reason to believe after reasonable enquiry that the deceased had expressed an objection to such a procedure, and that the surviving spouse or relatives do not object.

Removal must be by a fully registered medical practitioner who has satisfied himself that life is extinct. No tissues may be removed if there is reason to think that the death should be reported to the Coroner or the Procurator Fiscal.

Recently modifications of this procedure have been proposed, in Bills put before Parliament, to allow a medical practitioner to authorise removal of organs if the deceased has registered his consent in a register maintained by the Secretary of State.

Post-mortem examinations

Such an examination may be authorised by the person lawfully in possession of the body, provided that:

1 The Coroner or the Procurator Fiscal does not require to investigate the death.

2 Reasonable enquiry has shown that the deceased or any surviving relative has not objected.

Such examination may be performed by a fully registered medical practitioner or, on his instructions, by a provisionally registered practitioner or medical student.

Exhumation

This may be to allow removal of a body to another burial ground, and authorisation is then given by the ecclesiastical authorities. Exhumation for other reasons is normally authorised by a licence from the Home Office or may be by a Coroner's order. This may occur, for instance, when a death which has been certified as being due to natural causes appears on subsequent information to have been due to poisoning. In Scotland the Sheriff will authorise exhumation when appropriate, after receiving a request from the Procurator Fiscal.

Dying declarations

On occasions a patient dying as a result of a criminal act may yet be able to make a statement about the events, which will be able to be used at any subsequent trial, and the doctor should assist the person to give such evidence. However, certain rules must be obeyed for the statement to be valid.

1 The patient must be aware that he is dying, and that *he has no hope of recovery*, and must state this in the declaration.

2 The precise words of the patient must be recorded, if possible in writing at the time and signed by the patient, though an oral statement may be acceptable, recorded in writing as soon as practicable.

3 The patient must not be suffering from mental confusion.

4 The matter of the statement must only concern the circumstances responsible for the patient's approaching death.

Dying depositions

If a person is dangerously ill and unlikely to recover, a magistrate may take evidence on oath from him, and such a deposition may be used subsequently at a trial as evidence, if the patient has died or is too ill ever to attend court. Since there is opportunity for full cross-examination the deposition may relate to subjects other than the cause of the patient's illness or death.

Chapter 3
Medico-Legal Aspects of
Mental Disease

The purpose of this chapter is to outline the legal provisions for safeguarding the person and property of people suffering from mental disorder, or protecting the public, and to indicate how a person's disordered mental state may affect his responsibility under civil and criminal law. It does not deal with the clinical aspects of psychiatry.

Before 1890 there were few legal provisions for safeguarding the interests of mentally ill persons. However, the Lunacy Act of 1890, which was the principal Act until 1959, established, among other things, the procedure for compulsory admission of patients to mental hospitals after examination by a Justice of the Peace, if the patient was certified as being of unsound mind by a medical practitioner.

Provision for voluntary admission of a patient was first made by the Mental Treatment Act of 1930.

Mental Health Act s 1959–1983

This Act replaced the older statutes, in the light of the modern views on the medical treatment of mental illness. Only certain parts of the Act are considered here. For full details the Act itself or the various pamphlets issued by the Ministry of Health should be consulted.

A very recent piece of legislation, the Mental Health (Amendment) Act 1982 has modified some of the provisions of the Act of 1959, and is now consolidated in the Mental Health Act 1983.

In Scotland the relevant act is the Mental Health (Scotland) Act 1960. The principal differences from the English procedure are the setting up of a Mental Welfare Commission; and the method for compulsory detention in a mental hospital, where the application and supporting medical certificates are subject to the approval of the Sheriff after such inquiries as he thinks fit.

Classification of mental disorder

The Act defines certain classes of mental disorder. These are important since they affect the provisions made for patients.

Mental disorder—mental illness, arrested or incomplete development of the mind, psychopathic disorder, and any other disorder or disability of mind.

Mental illness—this is not defined by the Act which, however, refers to gross disturbance of thought, experience and behaviour arising as a new process in a person not previously manifesting such abnormality.

Severe mental impairment—a state of arrested or incomplete development of mind which includes severe impairment of intelligence and social functioning and is associated with abnormally aggressive or seriously irresponsible conduct on the part of the person concerned.

Mental impairment—means a state of arrested or incomplete development of mind (not amounting to severe mental impairment) which includes significant impairment of intelligence and social functioning and is associated with abnormally aggressive or seriously irresponsible conduct on the part of the person concerned.

Psychopathic disorder—means a persistent disorder or disability of mind (whether or not including significant impairment of intelligence) which results in abnormally aggressive or seriously irresponsible conduct on the part of the person concerned.

Admission to hospital

Informal (voluntary) admission
This is intended to be the principal means by which patients shall be admitted, whenever possible.

Compulsory admission
These provisions are intended to be used if the patient is suffering from a mental disorder which warrants his detention for assessment or treatment, and he is a danger to himself or others.

Admission for assessment (Sect. 25). A patient may be compulsorily admitted for assessment for a period not exceeding 28 days. The application may be made by the nearest relative or a social worker, who must have seen the patient within 14 days prior to the application. The social worker is contacted through the local division of the Department of Social Services.

The application must be supported by written recommendations of two doctors, one of whom must have special experience of mental disorder, while the other will usually be the patient's regular medical attendant. The recommendations need not indicate the precise nature of the mental disorder, but must state that compulsory detention is necessary in the interests of the patient, or others. The recommendations must be given before the application is made, and neither doctor may make the application himself, or be related to the applicant. The patient may be discharged from hospital by the responsible Medical Officer (usually the consultant in charge of the case) before 28 days have expired. If the patient is still in hospital after 28 days he may continue to stay as an informal patient or, in the event of continuing severe mental disorder Sect. 3 of the Act may be applied which will then ensure his compulsory stay in the hospital for a longer period.

Admission for treatment (Sect. 3). Such an application may be made in respect of a patient of any age suffering from mental illness or severe mental impairment, psychopathic disorder or mental impairment of a nature or degree making hospital treatment appropriate; that in the case of psychopathic disorder or mental impairment the treatment is likely to alleviate or prevent a deterioration in the condition; and that such detention for treatment is necessary for the health or safety of the patient or the protection of others.

The applicant may be the nearest relative or the social worker, but the latter may not make such application if the nearest relative objects.

Two medical recommendations are required, as in the case of admission for assessment, but in this case they must specify the nature of the illness, on which they must be in agreement, and indicate that other methods of treatment are not suitable.

Admission is initially for 6 months, and may be renewed subsequently at 1-yearly intervals.

Admission for assessment in an emergency (Sect. 4). In such a case application may be made by the nearest relative, or by the social worker. It is supported by one medical recommendation, usually by the regular medical attendant. However any qualified medical officer, such as a casualty officer, may make it. The applicant must have seen the patient within 24 hours prior to making the application.

Such an emergency admission may only be for 72 hours, but during this time the formalities may be completed for admission for assessment for 28 days.

Provisions also exist (Sect. 136) for removal of a mentally-ill person by a police officer to a 'place of safety', such as a mental hospital, where the person may be detained for up to 72 hours.

Compulsory reception into guardianship

Guardianship means the care of a patient over the age of 16 years, outside hospital, by some person or, more usually, the local authority. The guardian has powers in relation to the patient as to where he resides, to require him to attend for treatment, occupation, etc., and to ensure that access to the patient is provided for doctors and social workers.

Applications are in general similar to those for compulsory admission to hospital, and must be supported by two medical recommendations. The patient under guardianship must be visited regularly by a nominated medical practitioner. The guardianship is initially for 6 months, and may be renewed for 1 year at a time.

Discharge of patients

An order for discharge of a patient may be made by the hospital or local authorities, and may also be made by the nearest relative. The relative ordering discharge must give 72 hours' notice to the authorities, and discharge may be prevented if during this time the responsible medical officer makes a report stating that the patient would be likely to behave dangerously if discharged.

Leave of absence

Patients under compulsory detention may be granted leave of absence by a responsible medical officer. If absent without leave they may be taken into custody and returned to the hospital, by any social worker, officer of the hospital, or constable, unless they have been absent for more than 28 days.

Mental health review tribunals

These are appointed for each Regional Hospital Area by the Lord Chancellor. The members are chosen from the legal profession, the medical profession, or are persons having experience of administrative or social welfare work. A tribunal must contain one member from each of these groups.

The function of the Tribunal is to consider appeals against guardianship or compulsory detention in hospital from patients or relatives, and it may direct the discharge of a patient whom it considers is not suffering from mental illness at the present, or if further detention is considered to be unnecessary.

Provision for mentally ill patients charged with criminal offences

Compulsory admission to hospital or guardianship (Sect. 37). A Magistrate's Court or a Crown Court on convicting a person of any offence, other than murder, punishable with imprisonment, may order his compulsory admission to hospital or guardianship if:

1 Oral or written evidence of two doctors, one of whom has special experience of mental disorder, shows that the offender is suffering from

mental illness, psychopathic disorder, mental impairment or severe mental impairment of a nature or degree which warrants detention of the patient.

2 In the circumstances such detention is the best method of dealing with the case.

3 A hospital or guardian can receive the person.

A patient who has been admitted to hospital or guardianship on a court order is treated as though he has been compulsorily admitted for treatment, or received into guardianship in the usual way, except that his discharge may not be ordered by the nearest relative. On appeal the Mental Health Review Tribunal may order the patient's discharge.

If a person is convicted of an offence punishable with imprisonment, but is shown by medical evidence to be suffering from mental disorder the court may issue an interim hospital order, which is in force for up to 12 weeks, after which the court may decide what is the most appropriate mode of further disposal of the offender.

A court may also deal with a person who is accused, rather than convicted, by remanding him to hospital for a report on his mental condition, or remanding him for hospital treatment.

Restriction order (Sect. 41). Such an order may be made by a Crown Court, if it is considered necessary for the protection of the public from serious harm. Before such an order is made at least one doctor must give oral evidence relating to the offender's mental state.

A Magistrate's Court may not impose such an order. If it seems necessary to restrict the patient's discharge, the case must be referred to a higher court.

If such an order is imposed only the Home Secretary may authorise leave of absence or the discharge of the patient. The patient may ask that his case be referred by the Home Secretary to the Mental Health Review Tribunal.

Consent to treatment

The Mental Health (Amendment) Act 1982 specifies that with regard to certain forms of mental treatment specified by the Secretary of State, such as surgical treatment for destroying brain tissue, it is necessary first to obtain the patient's consent. This consent has to be supported by certificates from a medical practitioner and two lay persons that the patient can understand the implications of the treatment, and that it is appropriate to the patient's condition.

Such consent is not necessary for any treatment given in special circumstances, such as to save the patient's life, or where it is immediately necessary to prevent the patient behaving violently or being a danger to himself or others.

Care of a mental patient's property

A court known as the Court of Protection exists for this purpose, with a Master and Deputy Master who are appointed by the Lord Chancellor. A judge of the court, having heard medical evidence to show that a patient's mental state prevents him from managing his own affairs, may make such directions as are necessary to control the patient's property or carry on his business, or, more commonly, may appoint a receiver to attend to such matters.

The court can authorise the execution of a will on the patient's behalf; it will then require medical proof that the patient lacks testamentary capacity.

Certain legal and medical practitioners, who are appointed by the Lord Chancellor and are known as the Lord Chancellor's Visitors, have the responsibility of visiting such patients periodically and reporting to the judge on the patient's ability to manage his own affairs. The medical Visitor may require to examine the patient or to see any medical documents relating to the case, which may be in the possession of the patient's usual medical attendants.

Civil responsibility of mental patients

Contracts

A contract which has been entered into may be binding on the parties even though one party suffers from mental illness, unless it can be shown that the patient was incapable of understanding the contract and the other party knew of his mental illness, i.e. had perpetrated a fraud.

Torts, i.e. civil wrongs

A person is held to be responsible for his actions provided that he knows their nature and quality, and in such a case may be sued for damages.

Marriage

In the contract of marriage mental illness may be a ground for declaring the marriage null, or for divorce (see Chapter 4).

Witness

A person, even though suffering from mental illness, may be considered capable of giving valid evidence if the Court decides that the person is capable of understanding the significance of the oath and the necessity of telling the truth, and can make a coherent statement of the facts of a matter.

Making a will—testamentary capacity

A doctor may be required to examine a person suffering from mental disorder who wishes to make a will, in order to ascertain whether his mental state will permit a reasoned disposal of his property. Subsequently the doctor may be required to give evidence in court if the will is contested. A doctor would be well advised not to witness a patient's will unless he is prepared to testify later to the person's testamentary capacity, and as a witness he will forgo any legacy which he might have received from the will.

In deciding the capacity of the patient to make a will, the points which the doctor should consider are:

1   Does the patient realise he is making a will?
2   Does he know what property he possesses?
3   Does he understand which people have reasonable grounds for benefiting by the will?
4   Does he suffer from delusions which will cause unreasonable decisions?

Criminal responsibility of mental patients

If a person has committed a crime, notably homicide, his responsibility for his act, and the punishment to which he may be liable, can be modified to varying degree by the existence of mental illness, either at the time of the act or afterwards, for example:

Not guilty by reason of insanity

This is the modern version of the old verdict of 'guilty but insane', amended by the Criminal Justice Act 1948. It is based on the M'Naghten Rules of 1843, which were framed by a panel of judges after the trial of a man who, while suffering from a mental illness, shot and killed the secretary of Sir Robert Peel. Basically these state:

1   Every man is presumed sane and responsible for his acts until the contrary is proved.
2   To establish the defence it must be proved that at the time of the act the accused, by reason of disease of the mind, did not know what he was doing, or if he knew what he was doing then he did not know that it was wrong. These Rules do not apply in Scotland, as they have never been part of Scottish law.

Diminished responsibility

This defence was established by the Homicide Act 1957, to cover cases where, although the accused was not insane to a degree necessary to come within the M'Naghten Rules, yet his mental responsibility for his act was substantially impaired by some abnormality of mind, such as arrested or retarded development or conditions caused by disease or injury. Diminished responsibility has been an established part of Scottish law for a very long time.

In such a case, the accused's action in killing another is reduced from murder to manslaughter.

Other cases

Unfit to plead. If an accused is sent for trial at a Crown Court the defence may attempt to prove that the prisoner is suffering from mental disturbance to the extent of being unfit to be tried. This is based on medical evidence that the prisoner is unable to understand the nature of the evidence, to instruct his counsel or to follow the procedure of the trial. If the jury is satisfied on these points the prisoner, without standing trial, will be sent to Broadmoor or some other mental hospital.

Insane after conviction. If a patient is considered to be insane after he has been convicted of an offence, he may be dealt with under the appropriate sections of the Mental Health Act 1959 or Mental Health (Scotland) Act 1960, or the Home Secretary or Secretary of State for Scotland may order a special inquiry into the prisoner's mental state.

Chapter 4
Medico-Legal Aspects of Marriage, Divorce and Disputed Paternity

Impotence

This is the inability of a person to satisfy sexual desire in another, i.e. to have sexual intercourse, and may constitute a ground for nullity of marriage. It is not the same as sterility; a person may be unable to have children but may be quite capable of achieving sexual intercourse.

Impotence may be temporary or permanent, and may be due to age, general or local illness, or deformity of the sexual organs. Medical examination to determine the presence of such a condition may be required in cases of nullity of marriage or alleged rape.

Sterility

This does not constitute grounds for nullity of marriage or divorce.

Sterilisation by means of voluntary vasectomy is now legal (National Health Service (Family Planning) Amendment Act 1972).

Artificial insemination by the husband (AIH) is an ethically acceptable procedure for dealing with sterility. Artificial insemination by a donor (AID) is now a recognised procedure. Legitimacy of the child is established by the Family Law Reform Act 1987 (in England and Wales).

Nullity

A marriage may be declared null and void by the Courts on various grounds. Basically these show that either (a) one or other of the persons was incapable of being a party to a contract, e.g. from mental disorder, or (b) had in effect perpetrated a fraud, e.g. by being pregnant by someone else at the time of the marriage, or by being incapable of ever carrying out the requirements of the marriage contract, as by being impotent.

The principal grounds for a declaration of nullity of marriage are as follows:

1 Incapacity, or impotence. This is when the marriage cannot be consummated, i.e. it is impossible for there to be full penetration of the vagina by the penis, either from physical or mental disease, or deformity which cannot be corrected. Doctors will be required by the Court to examine both the husband and the wife to determine whether there is in fact any bar to the consummation of the marriage.

2 If one or other party deliberately refuses to consummate the marriage. Obstinacy, hysteria, frigidity, vaginismus, etc., may cause such a situation.

3 If a person, at the time of their marriage, was suffering from mental disorder so as to render them unfit for marriage, or was suffering from recurrent attacks of insanity or epilepsy.

4 If one of the parties was, at the time of the marriage, suffering from venereal disease in a communicable form.

5 When the wife, at the time of the marriage, was pregnant by a man other than the husband.

If a decree of nullity is sought on the grounds mentioned in paragraphs 3, 4 or 5 above, the petitioner must have been ignorant of the facts at the time of marriage, must institute proceedings within a year of the marriage, and must not have consented to marital intercourse since discovering the facts.

A marriage may also be declared void because of some 'administrative irregularity' such as the existence of a prior marriage of one of the parties, marriage within the prohibited degrees etc. These matters are not likely to require medical evidence.

Divorce

The sole ground for a petition for divorce, under the Divorce Reform Act 1969, is that the marriage has broken down irretrievably.

Proof of breakdown of the marriage may be that:

1 The respondent has committed adultery and the petitioner finds it intolerable to live with the respondent. Adultery occurs when one of the parties has voluntary sexual intercourse with someone other than the spouse. The doctor is rarely required, or indeed is able, by physical examination to prove that a married person has had extramarital intercourse. However, it may be alleged that a child born to the wife could not have been fathered by the husband. The grounds for such an allegation may be that the duration of pregnancy indicates that conception must have occurred at a time when the husband could not have had intercourse with the wife, e.g. if he was in another country. Alternatively, blood group determination may show that the husband could not be the father of the child (see below).

2 The respondent has behaved in such a way that the petitioner cannot reasonably be expected to live with the respondent. This corresponds to the old grounds for divorce of 'cruelty'. A doctor may be required to give evidence of injuries inflicted on the petitioner before the divorce proceedings were commenced, or to interpret injuries to general health, such as insomnia or weight loss.

3 The respondent has deserted the petitioner for a continuous period of at least 2 years immediately preceding the presentation of the petition.

4 The married couple have lived apart continuously for 2 years and both parties agree to the divorce.

5 The couple have lived apart for a continuous period of at least 5 years.

The last three matters are unlikely to involve a doctor, except in the case of mental illness of one of the parties.

Pregnancy

It may be important on certain occasions for the Courts to have medical evidence that a woman is pregnant, though a woman cannot be compelled to submit to examination for such a purpose.

1   A woman convicted of a capital offence. Formerly pregnancy constituted a bar to execution, though of course it is exceedingly unlikely that any woman will be in danger of execution in the future.

2   The fact that a woman is pregnant may affect the disposal of property by a will, since the unborn child may have a claim on the estate.

3   In cases of alleged abortion or concealment of birth, or in cases of libel or slander, where a woman has been accused of illicit sexual intercourse. Actions for breach of promise no longer exist, and so a doctor should beware of becoming involved in such disputes.

Signs of pregnancy

These are all dealt with in textbooks of obstetrics. To summarise, they are:

1   Presumptive:
Cessation of menstruation
Morning sickness
Breast changes
Abdominal enlargement
Hegar's sign
Uterine contractions.

2   Conclusive:
Foetal movement
Foetal heart sounds
X-ray demonstration of foetal structures
Biological tests.

Period of gestation

This may be of importance in cases of alleged adultery. The normal period is approximately 280 days, or 40 weeks. Living children can of course be born at 6 or 7 months of gestation, though they are then obviously immature. Conversely, a pregnancy may be protracted, and since courts are loath to pronounce a child illegitimate, durations of pregnancy of 331 days and up to 349 days have been accepted, but a duration of 360 days rejected.

Where a husband is shown to have had access to his wife, i.e. has been able to have sexual intercourse with her, as by being in the same house, and the child is born after a reasonable subsequent period of gestation, it will be taken to be his child, by the courts, unless illegitimacy can be proved by some other means, such as blood group determination.

Delivery

Medical evidence of recent delivery in a person may be sought in cases of alleged abortion or infanticide, or concealment of birth, and in disputed legitimacy of an offspring, e.g. when it is alleged that a woman has 'borrowed' an infant, and has pretended to have given birth to it, in order to gain some financial or social benefit, by fraud.

Signs of recent delivery are only summarised here, but details should be sought in obstetric textbooks.

1 Breast changes — production of milk.
2 Abdominal striae gravidarum.
3 Enlargement of uterus, softening of cervix, recent damage to perineum. Lochia.
4 Biological pregnancy tests.

Disputed paternity

This may arise in various circumstances, for example:

1 A married man may allege that his wife has committed adultery, and that he is not the father of a child which she has borne.

2 An unmarried girl who has an illegitimate offspring may allege that a certain man is the father of the child, in order to obtain an affiliation order against him.

In either event, the Court may seek medical assistance in determining the paternity of the child.

Such evidence may be called regarding the duration of pregnancy, as to whether it is consistent with conception having occurred at a time when the husband had access to his wife.

On occasions proof of parentage may be accepted on the grounds of close physical resemblance of the child to the alleged father, but such resemblance would have to be striking, such as distinctive colouring, or the presence in both parent and child of an obvious congenital deformity such as a supernumerary digit.

The use of blood group determination as a means of excluding a certain person as the parent of the child has a more reliable scientific basis, and is becoming increasingly used in the Courts; under the provisions of the Family Law Reform Act 1969, a court may direct that blood tests be used, if one of the parties to the proceedings applies. Samples of blood cannot be taken from any person without consent, but in the case of refusal the court may draw the appropriate inference. This Act does not apply to Scotland.

Blood group determination

The various human blood groups are known to be factors which are inherited on the lines established by Mendelian principles. Thus they provide a means of indicating the possible parentage of a child, since they are inherited characters which are easily determined.

The basic facts which make the blood groups of value in this field are (a) that a person's blood group remains constant throughout his life, except for transient disturbances after transfusion, and (b) that a person's blood group must be inherited from his or her parents, so that he cannot have a group which is not possessed by either of the parents (except in the very rare event of spontaneous mutation).

On Mendelian principles a person inherits one gene for each blood group from each parent, who themselves may be homo or heterozygous for the particular group. Thus in a blood group with several factors the result may be complicated. The principles may be demonstrated by considering the ABO group, for example:

		Group
(a) Mother		A (genotype AO)
Child		O
Possible fathers	1	B (genotype BO)
	2	A (genotype AO)
	3	O
	4	AB impossible—no O gene
(b) Mother		A
Child		AB
Possible fathers	1	B or AB possible
	2	A impossible—no B gene
	3	O impossible—no B gene

The same principles may be used for other blood group systems, of which the most commonly used after the ABO system are the rhesus and the MNS systems, following the same general principles.

Blood grouping cannot identify any particular person as the father of a child. Thus grouping may show that the child's father must be group B, but will not show which of the many people possessing group B blood. On the other hand the blood grouping may serve to exclude one particular person as the father, and this exclusion is the value of the method. The chance of exclusion of a person who is not the father is 18% using the ABO system. Obviously the more blood group systems which are tested independently then the greater the chance of exclusion, e.g. the best chance of an innocent man being excluded nowadays is about 90% using various serum groups and enzyme systems, as well as the ordinary blood groups.

Taking blood samples

Regulations under the Family Law Reform Act give details of how blood samples should be taken. A direction form as specified in the Regulations is sent to the doctor by the Court.

There is provision in the form for a photograph of the person from whom the Court has directed the sample to be taken, a declaration that the subject has not received a blood transfusion recently and forms of consent from the subject, or, if the subject is under a disability (e.g. a young child), the person having care of the subject. The form of the report of the person making the blood tests is also specified, and a scale of fees laid down.

Sufficient blood may be obtained from an infant by a heel prick, but it is preferable to delay the testing of the infant until it has reached the age of 1 year, as before this time the agglutinins (anti-A and anti-B) will not have developed.

Therapeutic abortion

The termination of pregnancy on medical grounds has become lawful, subject to the provisions of the Abortion Act 1967. Before the enactment of this statute, medical practitioners acting in good faith had to rely for protection from prosecution on decisions made in the Courts, notably R. v. Bourne 1939, which established precedents but were not binding on other Courts.

The main provisions of the Abortion Act are that termination of pregnancy is lawful when carried out by a registered medical practitioner, provided that two registered medical practitioners are of the opinion, formed in good faith:

1   That the continuance of the pregnancy would involve risk to the life of the pregnant woman or of injury to the physical or mental health of the pregnant woman or any existing children in her family greater than if the pregnancy were terminated; or

2   That there is a substantial risk that if the child were born it would suffer from such physical or mental abnormalities as to be seriously handicapped.

In determining whether the continuance of a pregnancy would involve such risk of injury to health as is mentioned in point 1 account may be taken of the pregnant woman's actual or reasonably foreseeable environment.

Termination must be carried out in a NHS hospital, or a hospital approved for this purpose by the Minister of Health or the Secretary of State.

A registered medical practitioner may terminate a pregnancy, even though the opinion of two registered medical practitioners is not available and the termination is not to be performed in a NHS or approved hospital, provided that in the particular case he is of the opinion, formed in good faith, that the termination is immediately necessary to save the life or to prevent grave permanent injury to the physical or mental health of the pregnant woman.

No person can be compelled to participate in any treatment authorised by this Act, if he has a conscientious objection; but this does not affect a duty to participate in treatment which is necessary to save the life or prevent grave permanent injury to the physical or mental health of a pregnant woman.

The Abortion Regulations 1968 set the form of certificate to be used by doctors when certifying that in their opinions an abortion is indicated and also require, in a prescribed form, the notification of the abortion to the Chief Medical Officer.

Chapter 5
Consent

A doctor does not have an automatic right to submit anyone to a medical examination or treatment. A physical examination, if conducted without the consent of the patient, could constitute in law (a) a criminal offence, an assault, either common or indecent, depending on the type of examination, or (b) a trespass upon the person. Therefore, it is important that the doctor should understand the different forms of consent, and also the circumstances in which each would be appropriate.

Occasions when consent is not required

1 On admission to HM Prison—for routine examination.
2 On a court order, of a person suffering from a notifiable disease or tuberculosis.
3 On the probation order of a court.
4 Of immigrants at ports and airports.
5 Of milk or food handlers.
6 Of school children, in state schools.

Thus all these cases are where refusal to allow examination might jeopardise the health of the community as a whole, or a substantial portion of it. In all other cases consent is necessary to medical examination.

Validity of consent

For a person's consent to be valid it must be genuine and freely given. He must understand what he is consenting to, and within reason what any possible results or complications might be. This is known as 'informed' consent, and its alleged lack is increasingly grounds for legal action against doctors. For instance a substantial amount of litigation has developed in cases of pregnancy of a partner following a vasectomy; it is alleged that doctors have failed to fully explain the effects of the operation and the possibility of failure to achieve sterility.

Therefore the doctor should take care to ensure that any procedures are explained to the patient and this fact is recorded in the clinical notes; this is particularly important with regard to complex modern methods of treatment, or participation in clinical trials. In such cases a senior doctor should give the explanation and countersign the consent form.

The consent must not be obtained by any sharp practice or blackmail, such as making some action of the doctor dependent on the consent of the person to some other procedure. Consent obtained by force, or fear, or fraud is always invalid.

The fact of consent when appropriate must be clearly stated. The fact that the patient does not say no, or obeys without saying anything, does not indicate consent

It is especially important to remember to ensure that consent is valid when dealing with persons suspected or accused of having committed some criminal offence.

Forms of consent

Implied

Implied by the behaviour of the patient. Thus the fact that a patient attends the surgery or summons the doctor to his house, complaining of illness, implies that he consents to a general physical examination, to determine the nature of the ailment. This implied consent is sufficient for all normal medical practice, but not if intimate examinations are to be made, e.g. rectal or vaginal examinations.

Express

Specifically stated by the patient either orally or in writing.

Oral consent. Where possible this should be given in the presence of a third party, otherwise the doctor has no proof of its existence if subsequently challenged. Oral consent should be sought before any of the intimate examinations, rectal or vaginal, before the performance of procedures such as a gastric test meal, or the taking of blood samples. A third person who is a disinterested party, i.e. not a friend or relative of the patient, should be present when an intimate examination is made to protect the doctor from subsequent accusations of indecent assault.

Written consent. This is necessary for the major procedures such as the administration of anaesthetics or the performance of operations. It is also necessary for examinations of persons accused of criminal offences. The protection societies have indicated the ideal consent form to be used in hospital, which makes it clear that the nature of the procedure and any complications have been explained to the patient, who also understands that the procedure is not to be carried out by any particular doctor

Valid consent cannot be obtained for a procedure which is illegal, such as euthanasia.

Consent in special cases

Normally consent as described above is given by the person concerned. However, this may not be possible, or may need to be qualified.

By a spouse

In operations interfering with marital rights, such as abortion or sterilisation, the consent of the patient is paramount, but the consent of the spouse should also be sought, though this cannot override the wishes of the patient. If the patient is unconscious or otherwise unable to give valid consent, then the consent of the spouse will be valid. Forms appropriate to the special circumstances have been prepared by the protection societies.

Minors (under 16 years of age)

The consent of the parent or guardian is necessary. If neither is available then the consent of the person in *loco parentis,* e.g. the headmaster of the child's school, is valid, in an emergency.

On occasions, parents may refuse permission for a procedure on their child which is necessary to save life, on religious grounds, e.g. blood transfusion is objectionable to Jehovah's Witnesses. It is possible then for a magistrate's court to order the child's removal from the care of the parents to that of a 'fit person', e.g. a county welfare officer, who may then give valid consent. However the Minister of Health has advised hospitals against adopting this procedure. Even if the doctor acts without consent, in such circumstances, provided that he does so in good faith to preserve the child's life, then he is unlikely to be in danger of legal action.

If a girl under 16 seeks contraceptive advice, it has been held to be lawful for a doctor to give such advice without parental consent, by the House of Lords, in the Gillick case. However the doctor should only do so if he can follow the guidelines set down in the judgement, or the GMC's 'Blue Book'.

Consent in emergency

If the patient is unconscious and no-one is available who could give consent, the doctor is entitled to carry out any procedures necessary to preserve life, but no more. Thus he may give blood transfusions, perform operations to relieve raised intra-cranial tension, etc. But a badly damaged limb, for instance, should not be amputated, provided that it does not constitute a danger to life, even if there is no doubt that subsequently it will be useless, without first obtaining the patient's consent.

Consent of mental patients

Under the provisions of the Mental Health (Amendment) Act 1982, it is necessary in certain circumstances to obtain the consent of a patient to specified treatment, in a particular form. For further details see Chapter 3.

Refusal of consent

In certain circumstances a patient may withhold consent to life-saving procedures. Thus a Jehovah's Witness who has been stabbed may refuse a blood transfusion, or a prisoner on hunger strike may refuse nourishment. Such situations put the doctor in considerable difficulties, and require him to consult his protection society, but in general it is advisable to respect the patient's wishes, even if this results in his death

There is currently much undecided argument about whether it is ethical, or lawful, to carry out testing for AIDS (acquired immune deficiency syndrome) on a blood sample without having obtained the patient's explicit consent for this procedure. The view expressed by the GMC is that consent must be obtained, except for some most exceptional circumstances.

Chapter 6
Negligence

Any citizen can be guilty of negligence. For a person to be judged negligent:

1 He must owe a duty to another person.
2 He must have committed a breach of that duty.
3 As a result the person to whom the duty was owed must have suffered some damage.

Translating this into terms of medical practice:

1 The person must be the doctor's patient, i.e. someone for whose medical care the doctor accepts responsibility.
2 The doctor must have done something which is not approved medical practice, or, more commonly, have omitted to do something which is considered accepted practice in the circumstances.
3 As a result of the action or omission the patient has suffered injury.

For example, a person attends casualty and is seen by the casualty officer (who accepts responsibility). He has suffered a fall on the hand which is painful, but no X-ray is taken and therefore no fracture diagnosed (omission of approved medical practice). Due to malunion of the fracture arthritis develops with incapacity of that hand (the patient has suffered damage).

When is duty owed?

This is from the moment that the doctor undertakes advice or treatment, whether under contract or gratuitously, e.g. at the scene of an accident. The doctor has no legal obligation to undertake the care of any patient, but once the obligation is accepted then he is liable to exercise proper skill and care in the management of the case.

Standard of duty

No doctor is expected to be perfect or infallible. The standard of competence which the patient is entitled to expect is that of an ordinary competent practitioner in the grade or speciality to which the doctor belongs. Thus the degree of skill expected in any one field of medicine is that of the average practitioner in that field. But a doctor would be ill-advised to go outside his sphere of competence. Thus a general practitioner performing major surgery will be expected to exercise the degree of skill of an average surgeon, unless he was forced to act in an emergency, when no surgeon was available.

Breaches of duty

Approved practice

If a doctor has followed approved medical practice, this will be taken as evidence of due care. Departure from approved practice, e.g. failure to take X-rays or to give antisera in appropriate circumstances is risky, leaving the doctor little defence if anything goes wrong. Doctors are expected to keep reasonably up to date by reading medical journals, but no-one is expected to read all the journals and be aware of all advances.

Accurate diagnosis

No doctor guarantees accuracy of diagnosis, and therefore cannot be considered negligent if an inaccurate diagnosis is made, unless it is shown that he did not exercise proper care in making it, e.g. failure to examine the abdomen of a child suffering from appendicitis, or failure to keep the child under observation if such a condition were suspected.

Risk of treatment

Some risks are inherent in any form of treatment and the doctor will not be negligent if they cause damage provided that he has taken reasonable care to avoid them, e.g. broken needle during injection. However, he may be negligent if he doesn't warn the patient beforehand of any appreciable risk involved, or inform him after a mishap has occurred.

Thus a needle would not be anticipated to break, and the patient need not be warned of the possibility. However, if it has broken then the patient should be told and arrangements made to remove the broken piece. If the doctor fails to notice that the needle has broken, or, having discovered this, does not tell the patient or make arrangements to prevent further damage, then he is negligent.

Communication with other doctors

Failure to inform a general practitioner of a person's discharge from hospital and treatment might constitute negligence if there was a reasonable possibility of some complication of the condition occurring. It has been held that such communication must be direct. To advise the patient to attend his own doctor or to give him a verbal message for the doctor in such circumstances is insufficient. This applies more to emergency treatment.

Attendance on patients

Failure to attend a private or NHS patient promptly when called may be held negligent when due to forgetfulness or laziness.

Res ipsa loquitor

This is a legal term meaning 'the thing speaks for itself'. Thus if after an operation the patient is found to have a swab or a pair of forceps left in the abdomen, this cannot be considered reasonable treatment, and the facts automatically indicate negligence. The onus then shifts to the doctor, to explain the facts if he can, or to show that the negligence was not his.

Such gross examples of negligence, such as swabs or instruments left in body cavities, transfusion of the wrong bottle of blood, amputation of the wrong limb, or performance of a certain operation on the wrong patient are the cause of various medical defence organisations paying out considerable sums of money in damages on behalf of their members each year. The facts are so obvious that it is usually impossible to defend the doctor, and settlements are made out of court. The prevention of these various catastrophes lies in careful identification, and rigorous checking procedures, for example, swab counts during an operation.

Medical records

When a doctor's standard of care is being disputed in an action for negligence, the principal evidence which he can produce in his defence is likely to be the medical records of the patient. Therefore it is important that these are carefully maintained. Moreover, following recent legislation, a Court may order their disclosure to 'the other side', and so it is important that derogatory or ill-founded comment about the patient is not included.

Criminal negligence

This is rare, and only occurs if the negligence is so gross that compensation is an inadequate redress and it constitutes a crime deserving punishment. This type of negligence is seen in a grossly careless act which results in death of a patient, as in obstetric delivery while drunk, or administration of an anaesthetic while under the effects of drugs. The doctor will then probably be charged with manslaughter and, upon conviction, may also be struck off the Medical Register.

Injury before birth

Following a Law Commission Report a new form of action has arisen in which a child can sue for injuries sustained before it was born, as for instance in a road accident to the pregnant mother (Congenital Disabilities (Civil Liability) Act 1976). However, it has been held by the Court of Appeal that a child born with disabilities cannot sue a doctor for failure to procure its abortion.

Nowadays many actions for negligence are based on allegations of failure to exercise due care when carrying out operations for sterilisation or abortion, with the result that the patient, or the spouse, becomes pregnant, or that the pregnancy proves not to have been terminated after all.

Medical defence societies

In any question of negligence the doctor would be well advised to consult his medical defence society before taking any action, in particular before making any admission. He should also remember that under the provisions of the Administration of Justice Act 1970, the Administration of Justice (Scotland) Act 1972 and Supreme Court Act 1981 the Court can compel the disclosure of a patient's medical records and so he should be careful to ensure that the records are complete, accurate, and do not contain any derogatory comments, exposure of which could be embarrasing for him.

Chapter 7
Professional Secrecy—Privileged Occasions

Normally a person is responsible for his statements and their consequences and may be sued for slander or libel, i.e. defamation of character. However, there are occasions when it may be necessary for a doctor as a duty to the public to make a statement which is derogatory. Then the doctor's statement is privileged if he acted in accordance with the rules, and he has a complete defence.

Usually any information received by a doctor from a patient is confidential and may not be disclosed to any other person. Obviously the doctor is allowed to disclose such information if the patient gives his consent. He may also have to disclose it in a court of law, when giving evidence; by law when issuing certain statutory certificates, such as death certificates and when notifying certain diseases; and when the safety of the community is paramount, as in the case of certain crimes.

Absolute privilege

This applies to any statements made in Parliament or in a court of law. No-one can be sued over any statements made in these places.

Qualified privilege

This provides protection against legal action when persons make statements in the course of their legal or social duty, but only if certain rules are observed:

1 The statement must not be malicious.
2 It must only be made to those having an interest or duty to receive it.

For example the statement on a death certificate that a person has suffered from syphilis is privileged, but the same statement made in conversation to a general member of the public is not protected and may result in legal action. Or, if a person is suffering from an infectious disease the doctor may need to inform the patient's employer, and would be protected against subsequent legal action, but not if the statement was also made to the patient's workmates. Thus a doctor must be very careful, when making statements about a patient, to whom he makes the statements.

Secrecy

At times there may be a difficult conflict between a doctor's duty to respect the confidence of his patient and to divulge information for the benefit of the community. Thus in the case of a motorist who is found to suffer epileptic attacks, it may be necessary to inform their employer or works medical officer, or the DVLC, if the patient refuses to disclose the facts. However regulations now permit the issue of a driving licence to an epileptic who has had no fits during the day for 3 years. The Road Traffic Act 1974 included a clause requiring drivers who became aware that they are suffering from a relevant disability to report this to the Secretary of State, and also if they have a prospective disability. The Secretary of State could then require the driver to authorise his doctor to release information about his disability to the licensing authority, who have a special section dealing with such information. Pregnancy in a girl under 16 years needs to be disclosed to the parents, but over 16 the girl's consent must be obtained first. A doctor was accused, though acquitted of serious professional misconduct for disclosing to her parents that a girl of 16 had been prescribed contraceptive pills by a clinic. The judgement in a recent case indicates that the request for contraceptive advice from a girl under 16 may be kept from the parents in certain circumstances (see p. 51).

Recent legislation has eroded secrecy in certain circumstances. In the case of a road traffic accident the law obliges a doctor to divulge information to the police, under the Road Traffic Act 1988; similarly the Prevention of Terrorism Act 1976 requires anyone with information which may lead to the apprehension of a person involved in an act of terrorism to inform the police; and for notification of drug addicts under the Misuse of Drugs Act (see p. 67). However, in all normal situations the doctor must take care to observe secrecy.

Medical documents

Nowadays it is especially important that doctors are aware of the hazards to confidentiality posed by the patients' medical records. If access to these is made too readily available, secrecy may be destroyed. Recent legislation has permitted a Court of Law to require disclosure of a patient's records to lawyers, for instance those acting for the patient in an action for negligence. Normally the requirement will be to release them to a medical practitioner acting on behalf of the lawyers. Certainly the doctor should not allow access to his patient's records by lawyers, police, or any other body, no matter how 'official' they may appear, in the absence of a Court order. Care should be taken even before releasing them to the patient's own solicitor, and the advice of the doctor's protection society sought. If the solicitor acts for a third party, such as employers, then the patient's consent is essential.

It must be remembered that any records held on computer are now subject to the Data Protection Act of 1984. Moreover, under the Access to Medical Reports Act 1988, patients can demand to see reports written about them for purposes of employment or insurance, can refuse to let the report be sent out, or add objections to it.

Chapter 8
Compensation

A person who suffers an injury as the result of an accident will usually be able to claim compensation. This may be by legal action in a civil court against the person responsible for the accident, or it may be a claim on the State under the National Insurance Acts.

In either event, a doctor is likely to be required to give evidence of the nature and consequences of the patient's injuries, and their relationship to the accident.

Medical precautions

It is as well for a doctor to remember that any injury which he is called upon to treat may later become the subject of a claim for compensation, and that such a claim, especially where civil law action is involved, may take a year or more before the stage is reached where the doctor's evidence is required. A legal control, under the Limitation Acts, is imposed to prevent unreasonable delay in commencing legal action for compensation for a personal injury. Such an action must usually be started within 3 years from the date of the injury, unless the injury is of a type which is only slowly manifested. In such a case the claimant must show that material facts of a decisive character relating to his injury were unknown to him until 3 years had elapsed, and that the action was started within 12 months of the discovery of those facts, and the leave of the court must be obtained. Even so by the time the legal procedure has reached the stage of a court hearing a doctor may find himself giving evidence about an event which occurred 4 or 5 years previously. Moreover, under the Limitation Act 1975, a court may overrule the 3 year period if it seems necessary in the interest of justice.

Therefore whenever he treats an injury, however trivial, he should remember the possibility of litigation at some time in the future, and should be particularly careful to make adequate notes of the nature of the injury and the treatment given and whether the patient's disability was or was not related to the accident. These he can refer to when called upon to give evidence many months later. If the injury is of any magnitude, and requires prolonged treatment, then the notes should contain assessments of the amount of pain, distress, etc. involved, since these may need to be considered later when a Court is assessing damages, and can only be estimated reliably by the doctor. Loss of earnings, and the impairment of abilities at the time of the claim can usually be assessed by the Court without the doctor's help, but he may be required to express an opinion as to the prognosis of any disability.

It is, of course, well known that conditions may be attributed by the patient to an injury, but without any foundation in fact. Also the degree of a person's disability may be considerably exaggerated by psychological disturbances of the patient, i.e. compensation neurosis, the condition being alleviated by settlement of the claim in the patient's favour. This is not the same as malingering, where the person deliberately falsifies symptoms and injuries for gain, financial or otherwise, but in either case the doctor must be ready to detect and take into account these conditions when giving opinions about the patient's disabilities.

In addition to treatment of a living patient, the doctor may be required to decide whether a person's death was a consequence of an accident or injury, or attributable to his work, since the dependants may then have grounds for claiming compensation.

The doctor must remember to preserve his confidential relationship with his patient. The consent of the patient should be obtained before disclosing information to an employer, especially of old medical records.

Relationship between trauma and disease

There are certain conditions which are well-recognised as being consequences of trauma, e.g. pulmonary embolism. There are others where the relationship is very debatable, and is usually denied, e.g. tumour formation, except in a few special circumstances. There is no doubt that this field of forensic medicine causes greater dispute than any other. Therefore it is important that the doctor should be cautious, should consider the facts very carefully before expressing an opinion, and should not diverge from accepted medical views unless he has very good reason. Carelessly considered opinions may lead to useless litigation, and to the doctor's discredit and embarrassment.

Examples of certain commonly queried relationships are given here, but obviously the list is by no means exhaustive, since the question of the relation between trauma and almost every known disease could be and probably has been raised.

Conditions commonly accepted as being a sequence to trauma

Venous thrombosis and pulmonary embolism

Deep vein thrombosis, especially in the legs, possibly associated with pulmonary embolism, is well-recognised as being related to an injury, if it occurs 1–2 weeks later, and following a period of immobility. Increased viscosity of the blood, platelet adhesiveness and venous stasis have been suggested as the predisposing factors.

Broncho-pneumonia

This commonly occurs in elderly people following a fracture with consequent immobility; the shock and the immobility with bad postural drainage are the probable causes.

Peptic ulcer

As an acute duodenal ulcer, known as Curling's ulcer, this may occur as a complication of burns or scalds, or of fractures; the mechanism is unknown.

Tumour

In the vast majority of cases it is considered that there is no reason for connecting trauma and tumour development. Experimental work has not revealed any tumour growth after a single injury. However, in some cases of meningiomas, the growth has been found to develop at the exact site of a previous cranial injury, especially a fractured skull as shown by Cushing; the mechanism may be sequestration of fragments of dura in the fracture line. Skin cancer is well recognised as a hazard of radiation. On other occasions, tumours, e.g. of bone, may occur within a few weeks or months of trauma, and in the absence of definite proof to the contrary, a Court is likely to take the view that it is probable that trauma has played a part either in initiating or accelerating the rate of growth of the tumour. There may, of course, be a clear connection between the tumour and the victim's work, e.g. a mesothelioma or a carcinoma of the bronchus, in an asbestos worker.

Conditions which may be aggravated by trauma

Coronary occlusion by atheroma

Sudden increased demands for blood by a heart with a deficient arterial supply due to coronary atherosclerosis, may precipitate a cardiac infarction with severe pain, or sudden collapse and death during the exertion. A coronary thrombosis, on the other hand, is rarely related to trauma, except in the uncommon instance when trauma to the chest causes damage to the coronary vessel, which is then followed by thrombosis. Sometimes it is associated with burns.

Rupture of aneurysms

Direct violence may occasionally cause rupture of an aneurysm, as for example when a forcible blow to the head causes sub-arachnoid haemorrhage from rupture of a 'berry' aneurysm of a cerebral artery. More commonly the rupture is held to be due to a rise in blood pressure which is a consequence of unaccustomed physical exertion.

Ewing's postulates

This set of criteria was suggested when considering the relationship between trauma and tumours. However, in general they are applicable in many other situations. It is suggested that in order to establish a probable relationship between an injury and a tumour:

1 The part of the body must have been quite healthy before the accident.
2 It must be proved that adequate trauma was applied to the part.
3 A tumour must have occurred within a reasonable time interval after the trauma.
4 The tumour must occur in the exact location of the trauma.
5 The nature of the tumour must be proved by microscopical examination.

In fact these postulates are an attempt to introduce some rationalism into the common assumption that two events which are closely related in time must be cause and effect. They do not provide very scientific proof of a relationship even when they are satisfied, but by considering them the doctor will often be able to clarify his views on a given situation.

Insurance

Private insurance

A doctor may be requested by an insurance company to make a medical examination of a proposer. It must be remembered that any false information given in a certificate of insurance will cause the policy to be void, and if a doctor deliberately gives false information he may be guilty of fraud and also liable to disciplinary action by the GMC. He must therefore be particularly careful to avoid being persuaded or misled into omitting or ignoring any tests or abnormal findings.

National Insurance

This provides sickness and unemployment insurance for all workers, and retirement pension, widow's pension, maternity grants, etc. Before a claimant can receive many of these benefits a doctor may be required to complete a medical certificate, notably in support of claims for sickness benefit; first, intermediate and final certificates being needed. The doctor should be very careful not to be coerced into issuing such certificates without being satisfied by personal examination that the claimant is in fact sick, i.e. not to issue certificates to a relative without seeing the patient. Such conduct would constitute issuing false certificates, and could lead to disciplinary action by the GMC.

Industrial injuries

The Social Security Acts 1975 and 1986 have replaced the National

Insurance (Industrial Injuries) Act 1946. The provisions, however, are basically unaltered.

By the provisions of this Act, employed persons are insured by a fund maintained by contributions from the workmen, the employers, and the State, against accidents and certain prescribed diseases occurring at work, or while travelling in connection with work. Such benefit, unlike a civil litigation claim, may be payable even though the injured person has disobeyed instructions or safety regulations and had sustained the injury as a consequence. The benefits consist of:

1 Statutory sick pay—during sickness after an accident.
2 Industrial disablement benefit—when a permanent disability results.
3 Industrial death benefit.

The claimant must:

1 Give notice of the accident as soon as possible.
2 Make claims in a standard form.
3 Submit to a medical examination, and to treatment and rehabilitation, if this is possible.

The claim, supported by appropriate certificates, goes first to the Insurance Officer. He may allow, or disallow the claim, or may refer it to the Local Appeal Tribunal. The claimant may also appeal to the Tribunal, and after that to the National Insurance Commissioner.

A person claiming disablement benefit is referred by the Insurance Officer to a Medical Board, consisting of two or more medical practitioners who assess his disability. The claimant may appeal against the Board's decision to a Medical Appeal Tribunal.

In addition to accidents, certain diseases, which are recognised as resulting from special forms of employment, are prescribed by the Act and persons in such employment who suffer from them are automatically entitled to benefit.

The diseases and the special forms of employment are listed in schedules to the Act, which should be consulted for full details. Examples of such diseases are:

1 Heat cataract from the frequent or prolonged exposure to the glare of molten glass or red-hot metal.
2 Infection by *Leptospira icterohaemorrhagica* from work in rat-infested places.
3 Lead poisoning from any occupation involving the use or handling of, or exposure to the fumes, dust or vapour of lead or its compounds.
4 Pneumoconiosis, in coal miners and quarry workers.

Chapter 9
Poisons Legislation

Control of poisons

Until recent times the sale of poisons was not subject to any legal control. The first attempt to institute such control was in 1851, when the Arsenic Act was passed. The first comprehensive legislation was the Pharmacy and Poisons Act 1933; the most recent is the Poisons Act 1972.

Poisons Act 1972

This Act is concerned principally with non-medicinal poisons.

A panel of experts, known as the Poisons Board, assist the Home Secretary to prepare a list of substances which should be considered to be poisons, requiring control. The Board also assists in making Poisons Rules, controlling the acquisition, storage, etc., of these substances. The objects of the Rules are to prevent unlawful acquisition of poisons, while at the same time allowing supplies to be obtained by persons having a legitimate reason, with the minimum of inconvenience. The Poisons List and Rules are revised and consolidated from time to time. They can be obtained from HMSO.

Poisons List

This contains all the non-medicinal substances which are considered to require restriction. The list is divided into two parts:

Part I contains substances such as hydrogen cyanide, which may only be sold by a person conducting a retail pharmacy business.

Part II contains substances, for instance formaldehyde, which may be sold by a person conducting a retail pharmacy business, or by a person whose name is entered in a local authority list, such as a proprietor of a horticultural shop.

Poison Rules

These impose specific restrictions on certain groups of poisons. The poisons are divided into 14 Schedules. These are mainly concerned with storage and transport of poisons.

The Rules only concern a doctor in so far as he may wish to purchase a non-medicinal poison like any other member of the public. In the case of any poison included in Schedule I of the Rules, such as paraquat, the purchaser must be known to the seller, or must produce a certificate signed by a householder that he may properly be supplied with the poison. The purchaser must also sign an entry in a 'poisons book', kept by the seller which contains details of the sale.

If a doctor requires a poison included in Schedule I for his profession, he may send a signed order, in writing, stating his name, address, profession, the purpose for which he requires the poison, and the total quantity to be purchased. The poison can be ordered by telephone, provided a signed order is delivered to the seller within the next 24 hours.

Control of medicines

Medicines Act 1968

The provisions of this Act deal mainly with the establishment of a Medicines Commission, with licences and certificates relating to the production of medicines, with pharmacies, and with the British Pharmacopoeia. However Part III relates to the sale or supply of medicinal products and to prescriptions.

Prescriptions

Under the earlier legislation, the Pharmacy and Poisons Act 1933, certain medicines were classed as Schedule 4 poisons and could only be sold on a prescription from a doctor, dentist, or veterinary surgeon. These medicines included such things as barbiturates and tranquillisers.

Under the new legislation these drugs, together with an additional list of medicines included in the Medicines (Prescription Only) Order 1977 can only be supplied on a prescription. All medicines for parenteral injection, except insulin, are 'prescription only'.

A valid prescription for a prescription only medicine:

1 Must be written in indelible ink.

2 Must contain the following particulars:

(a) the address and usual signature of the practitioner giving it;

(b) the date on which it was signed by the practitioner giving it;

(c) such particulars as indicate whether the practitioner giving it is a doctor, or a dentist, a veterinary surgeon or a veterinary practitioner;

(d) where the practitioner is a doctor or a dentist, the name, address, and the age (if under 12) of the person for whose treatment it is given.

3 Must not be dispensed later than 6 months after the date on which it was signed by the prescriber except where it is a repeat prescription (that is, a prescription which contains a direction that it may be dispensed a stated number of times).

4 Where it is a repeat prescription, must not be dispensed other than in accordance with the direction contained therein.

5 Where the prescription is not a repeat prescription but contains a direction that the prescription be repeated without specifying the number of

times it may be dispensed, must not be dispensed on more than two occasions unless it is a prescription for oral contraceptives in which case the prescription may be dispensed six times during the period of 6 months following the date specified in the prescription.

Emergency supply to patients

If, in an emergency a doctor cannot give a prescription at once to the patient, a pharmacist may supply a medicine provided that:

1   The pharmacist is satisfied that a doctor has requested the supply.

2   The doctor undertakes to furnish a prescription within 72 hours.

3   The medicine is supplied in accordance with the doctor's directions, but cannot be repeated.

4   That the medicine is not a drug in Schedule 2 of the Misuse of Drugs Act.

5   That an entry is made in an appropriate register.

OR

If a patient requests a POM (prescription only medicine) from a pharmacist, without having a prescription, the pharmacist may supply it providing that:

1   The pharmacist is satisfied that there is an immediate need for the medicine.

2   This medicine has been given to the patient before by a doctor.

3   The pharmacist is satisfied as to the appropriate dose.

4   Only sufficient medicine for 3 days treatment is supplied.

5   That the supply is recorded in an appropriate register.

6   That the drug is not in Schedule 2 of the Misuse of Drugs Act, or the Special Medicines List.

7   That the medicine is specially labelled.

Control of drug addiction

Previously this was complicated by the number of acts involved, notably the Dangerous Drugs Act. Now these have been consolidated and superseded by the Misuse of Drugs Acts 1971, which incorporates most of their features. This Act covers the following:

1   It sets up an advisory council, charged with keeping under review the situation in the United Kingdom with respect to drugs which are misused (principally drugs of addiction) and advising the Government on measures for their control.

2   The drugs affected by the Act are called 'controlled drugs'. There are three classes, i.e.

Class A (e.g. morphine)

Class B (e.g. cannabis)

Class C (e.g. methaqualone)

This classification is concerned with grading penalties for offences when drugs in different classes are involved. For instance the maximum penalty for an offence involving:

Class A drug: life imprisonment, for both trafficking and possession.

Class B drug: 5 years imprisonment for possession and 14 years for trafficking.

Class C drug: 2 years imprisonment for possession and 5 years for trafficking.

3 It is an offence to import or export controlled drugs, to supply them or to possess them, unless authorised (e.g. a doctor is authorised to possess and supply them).

4 The Home Secretary shall make regulations dealing with storage, prescriptions, etc.

5 If a doctor commits an offence under this Act, or if it appears that he has behaved irresponsibly with regard to prescribing or supply, etc., of controlled drugs, or has contravened regulations in respect of supplying or notifying addicts, the Home Secretary may issue a direction prohibiting the doctor from using those or any controlled drugs.

In the event of irresponsible behaviour or contravention of regulations the Home Secretary may refer the case to a tribunal set up under the Act to consider the matter. The tribunal will advise the Home Secretary whether to issue a direction or not. In an urgent case the Home Secretary may issue a temporary direction, after consulting a professional panel, and must then, while the temporary direction is in force, refer the case to a tribunal.

6 If a 'drug problem' appears to be occurring in a particular area, a doctor may be obliged to give details, of controlled drugs which he has supplied, on the request of the Home Secretary. Details of the patients concerned need not be divulged.

Misuse of Drugs Regulations 1985

Classification of drugs

The regulations make an additional classification of drugs, into Schedules, e.g.

Schedule 1 (e.g. cannabis and LSD)

Schedule 2 (e.g. morphine)

Schedule 3 (chlorphentamine and barbiturates)

Schedule 4 (e.g. diazepam)

Schedule 5 (e.g. codeine)

Drugs in Schedule 1 can only be used under a special licence from the Home Office. Only doctors and dentists may administer drugs in Schedules 2 and 3. Drugs in Schedule 4 are affected by the POM regulations of the Medicines Act, as are some of the drugs in Schedule 5.

Drugs in Schedules 2, 3 and 4

1   *Supply to doctor*. This may be by a 'signed order' or requisition in the same form as that described above, under the Poisons Act 1972. In an emergency the doctor may order a supply of drugs by telephone, provided he supplies a written requisition within 24 hours.

2   *Prescription*. Such a prescription may not be dictated by the doctor over the telephone, but in other respects is the same as the form of prescription described above for POM drugs under the Medicines Act. However, the doctor, as well as signing and dating the prescription himself, must also write the name and address of the patient and the total quantity and dose of the drugs. This prevents the issue of prescriptions by unqualified persons such as receptionists. A prescription can only be used to supply drugs to a particular patient. If the patient dies unused drugs must be destroyed, not re-used.

3   *Registers*. For drugs in Schedules 1 and 2, registers must be kept of drugs obtained and of drugs supplied or administered. There must be a separate part for each class of drugs. Entries must be made in chronological order, on the same day that the drug is obtained or supplied, or not later than the next day. The entries must be indelible, and no alteration or obliteration is allowed. The entry must indicate the date, name and address of supplier or person supplied, the authority of a person supplied to possess the drug, the amount of the drug and the form in which it was received or supplied. Loose-leaf books may not be used. If the doctor has more than one surgery, separate sets of records must be kept for each, and these records must be available for inspection at any time for a period up to 2 years from the date of the last entry. Sales of Schedule 2 drugs are recorded by the pharmacist in a Controlled Drugs Register.

Safe custody regulations

These apply to drugs in Schedules 1 and 2. The doctor must keep such drugs in a locked receptacle, which can be opened by him, or a person authorised by him. A locked car is not a 'locked receptacle'.

Notification of and supply to addicts regulations

An addict is defined as a person who, as a result of repeated administration has become so dependent upon the drug that he has an overpowering desire for the administration of it to be continued.

If a doctor attends a person whom he diagnoses as a drug addict he must, in the next 7 days, send in writing to the Chief Medical Officer at the Home Office details, e.g. name, address, NHS number. This does not apply if the doctor is satisfied that continued administration of drugs is needed for the treatment of organic disease or injury; or notification of the addict has been made within the last 12 months.

A doctor shall not supply to a drug addict any cocaine or heroin or dipi-panone, unless he is licensed by the Home Secretary to treat drug addicts, or else the drugs are needed to treat an organic disease or injury.

(For details of drug addiction *see* Chapter 30.)

Solvent abuse

Under the Solvent Abuse (Scotland) Act 1983 any child caught abusing solvents can be referred to a children's panel (equivalent to a juvenile court), and may be taken into care compulsorily. Control of sale in England is by the Intoxicating Substances (Supply) Act 1985.

Chapter 10
Court Procedure

Coroner's Court

The office of Coroner is an ancient one; certainly dating from the time of Richard I, possibly earlier. His original powers and duties were extensive, but today his function is mainly restricted to the investigation of obscure or unnatural death.

The Coroner is appointed by the local authority, but he can only be dismissed by the Lord Chancellor. He may be either a lawyer or a doctor of not less than 5 years' standing; the majority of Coroners are solicitors but certain Coroners, notably in London, are doubly qualified, in medicine and law.

Coroner's procedure

The Coroner is empowered to enquire into the cause and circumstances of any death, when the cause is obscure or apparently unnatural, and into the death of a prisoner.

Once the death has been notified to the Coroner, preliminary enquiries are made on his behalf by his officer. This officer is usually a serving police officer, seconded either whole-time, or only during the investigation of a particular case. The scene of death, and the body of the deceased, are viewed, statements taken from witnesses, and a police report is submitted to the Coroner. Usually a post-mortem examination of the deceased is performed by a pathologist, on the instructions of the Coroner.

If the result of the enquiry is to show that death is due to a natural cause, the Coroner will usually conclude the enquiry by issuing his 'Pink form' (Form 100 Part B), which is a certificate of cause of death, for the purpose of registration of the death. He may also issue an order for burial, or, if disposal is to be by cremation, Form E which replaces Forms B and C under the regulations of the Cremation Acts.

The Coroner is entitled to hold an inquest on any case which is reported to him, but in practice usually only does so when the cause of death is unnatural. In certain circumstances, e.g. death following a road traffic accident, or the death of a prisoner, he is obliged by law to hold an inquest.

Coroner's inquest

In large cities the Coroner has his own courtroom, but elsewhere he may conduct his inquest in any convenient place, other than licensed permises, e.g. a police station, hospital boardroom, Magistrate's Court, etc. The Coroner's Officer keeps order in the Court, marshals the witnesses, and may administer the oath to them.

A witness must take the oath, or affirm, according to his religious conviction. His evidence is given in the form of answers to questions put to him by the Coroner. Lawyers may attend the Court to represent interested parties, and may at the discretion of the Court question the witness, and the Coroner may also allow questions to be put by relatives, or the foreman of the jury. The witness must answer all questions put to him, except for those which, if answered, might force him to incriminate himself.

The medical practitioner usually required to give evidence at an inquest is the pathologist who performed the post-mortem examination, but any general practitioner or hospital doctor may find himself summoned to an inquest to give evidence about the death of one of his patients. Such a summons must be obeyed; failure to comply constitutes contempt of court. The doctor should take care to refresh his mind of the facts of the case before giving evidence. His attendance is never required as a mere formality. Also he should take with him all relevant documents which he possesses, e.g. medical records, X-rays, etc.

He must not be misled by the apparent informality of the proceedings, an impression liable to be fostered by the location of the inquest, and the fact that the Coroner and any lawyers present are not robed. He must give careful thought to the statements that he makes, because (a) they are made on oath, and deliberate falsehood is then perjury, and (b) the record of evidence (the deposition) may be relevant in any subsequent criminal or civil proceedings. Ill-considered opinions and statements made in the Coroner's Court may have far-reaching consequences, and may be the starting point of lengthy, costly, and pointless litigation.

After giving evidence, the doctor will usually be released by the Coroner, but may not leave the Court without such permission.

The Coroner's duty at his inquest is restricted to determining who the deceased was, when and where he died, and the cause of death. The power which he previously had to commit a person to the Crown Court on a charge of murder, manslaughter, or infanticide has been abolished by the Criminal Law Act 1977. Moreover he cannot consider or decide questions of civil liability. Therefore the possibility that a doctor has been negligent will not be considered in the Coroner's Court, though if the facts indicate criminal negligence the Coroner may refer the case to the Director of Public Prosecutions. Nevertheless, evidence given in the Court may form the basis for subsequent litigation at a civil court, and in such circumstances the doctor is entitled and would be well advised to be legally represented at the inquest.

The fees payable to witnesses are fixed by law (Coroners Fees and Allowances Rules).

Because **Scotland** has a separate legal system, an entirely different system of enquiring into deaths exists. Each town and district has a Procurator Fiscal, appointed by the Lord Advocate in Edinburgh, part of whose duties is to investigate sudden and unexpected deaths. Because he is always a lawyer, and not a medical practitioner, he will usually request an autopsy to be carried out. Strictly speaking, he is not interested in the precise cause of death, rather, his remit is to determine whether or not any criminality has taken place. If there is no evidence of criminality his interest usually ends there. If he wishes to have an autopsy he applies to the Sheriff of the area for a warrant to authorise one (or two) pathologists to carry it out.

The Fiscal's enquiries thereafter are conducted in private; he may separately precognose all the witnesses to the affair in his office, after which he will send his report to the Crown Office for senior lawyers to decide whether there is a case to answer and in what level court it should be decided. With regard to certain deaths the Fiscal *may* hold a public enquiry before a Sheriff, sitting without a jury. Certain deaths *must* be inquired into and often the Crown Office itself orders a public enquiry under the Fatal Accidents and Sudden Death Inquiry (Scotland) Act 1976.

The Procurator Fiscal leads the evidence and the Sheriff decides the outcome, unlike the English system where the Coroner plays both roles.

Magistrate's Court

In these courts the bulk of the minor criminal work is carried out, and also more serious cases proceeding to the Crown Court for trial are examined to ensure that there really is *prima facia* (i.e. an apparently genuine) case against the accused. The doctor may be required to give evidence in the Magistrate's Court at such preliminary hearings, or 'committals', and also in cases of alleged drunkenness, assault, sexual offences, etc.

The Court is presided over by one or more magistrates, or justices of the peace, who are not lawyers. They have a Clerk of the Court, a lawyer, to advise them on legal matters. Lawyers, who are usually solicitors, conduct the prosecution and the defence.

The doctor, when called, will take the oath, and will then be questioned first by the prosecuting solicitor. He will then be cross-examined by the defending solicitor, and may also be questioned by the magistrate, who should be addressed as 'Your Worship' or 'Sir'.

If the case in which the doctor is giving evidence is a 'committal', he must remember to speak slowly, as his evidence is being taken down as he speaks, usually on a typewriter, by the Clerk. When his evidence is concluded, this record, known as his deposition, will be read back to him and if it is correct he must sign it. Therefore he must be sure that it is a true record of his statements and opinions, as it will be used as the basis of his evidence at the higher Court, and departure from it there will cause adverse comment.

Crown Courts

As a result of the Courts Act 1971, these replaced the Quarter Sessions and Assize Courts. There are three tiers of Crown Courts, the first tier resembling the old Assize Courts in that the court can try criminal or civil cases, and is presided over by a High Court Judge.

All the more serious criminal cases except treason, e.g. murder, rape, robbery with violence, etc., are dealt with at Crown Courts, and are tried by a jury. Barristers conduct the prosecution and the defence, and are known as counsel.

A doctor may be called to give evidence by either the prosecution or the defence. His evidence will usually have been given earlier in statements to the police and in evidence given in the lower court (the Magistrate's Court) when the case was first heard at the committal stage, and that evidence forms the basis of his examination at the Court.

No matter which side calls him, it is important that the doctor gives his evidence in an impartial and objective manner, stating the facts clearly, and his conclusions drawn from them, without concern as to whether they favour one or other side. If he appears to be biased he will be liable to severe cross-examination, and his opinions will be suspect.

When warned to attend the Court to give evidence (the warning will probably only be given on the evening before the case is to be heard), the doctor would be well-advised to refresh his mind on the facts of the case, especially since the case will probably not come to trial until several months after the alleged crime was committed. For this reason it is also essential that the doctor should have accurate and reliable notes to which he may refer. On arriving at court the following day, the doctor should be prepared for a long wait, since the case may involve 10 or 20 witnesses, and may last for 2 days or even longer.

When called into Court the doctor should take with him into the witness box all the relevant notes, reports and X-rays of the case. He is allowed to refer in the box to reports and X-rays, and to notes made at the time of the examination, to refresh his memory. He will be questioned first by the counsel of the party which has called him. This is known as the examination-in-chief, and during this the relevant medical facts, and the conclusions which the doctor has drawn from these facts are elicited.

Next the counsel for the other party will cross-examine the doctor. He will ask questions designed to test whether any examination of tests, which might lead to a different interpretation of the case, have been omitted, and whether any alternative conclusions could be tenable on the facts. Finally the doctor may be re-examined by the first counsel, to clear up points which may have arisen during cross-examination. At any stage the Judge may interpose, to disallow a question for legal reasons, or to clarify a point. He must be addressed as 'My Lord'. If the doctor feels he cannot answer a question without betraying professional secrecy, then he should appeal to the Judge, and must act as he directs.

Barristers are courteous and correct, and provided that the doctor knows his facts, he need not fear their examination. He in his turn must be polite when answering questions, and be prepared to admit any alternative explanation of the facts which is reasonable, when put to him even if he had not thought of it.

He must be careful to speak slowly, so that he may be audible, and also to aid the shorthand writer, who has to make a record of all that is said. Whenever practicable he must also restrict himself to simple words and avoid technical terms and phrases, since the jury will not understand them. For instance it is better to describe an incised wound as a 'cut', or a metacarpo-phalangeal joint as a 'knuckle'.

When the doctor's evidence has been given, the counsel for the party who called the doctor will normally ask the Judge if the doctor may be released, to return to his practice. Whether the doctor does so, or has to remain in the Court, he should refrain from speaking to witnesses who have not yet given evidence, lest collusion be suggested.

Civil Courts

The majority of these are County Courts, and are presided over by County Court Judges, who are addressed as 'Your Honour'. These courts deal with all the relatively minor matters of civil litigation, the more serious cases going to the High Court. The form of the procedure is much the same as in the criminal courts. The advocates may be either solicitors or barristers. The doctor who is called to give evidence will be examined, cross-examined and re-examined in the same way as in the other courts. Questions of compensation and of negligence will come to such courts, and the medical evidence is likely to be more concerned with balance of probabilities than in the criminal courts, where proof is required. Therefore it is likely that each party will obtain the services of a doctor. In such an event it is important to avoid dispute and wrangling. The doctor should ensure that the views he expresses are in accord with the facts and should firmly but politely adhere to his conclusions.

At all times when giving evidence in any court the doctor should remember that his sole purpose is to aid the court in arriving at a just decision, by describing and explaining the medical aspects of the case, and the conclusions which can be drawn from them. Whether these support one or other side in a dispute should be quite immaterial to him.

He should remember that it is no disgrace to have to admit that he does not know the answer to any particular question, and that to admit this at once is infinitely preferable to being forced to admit ignorance after a prolonged attempt to evade the issue. Moreover he should never attempt to answer questions on subjects which are outside his sphere of competence.

In **Scotland**, the overall structure is similar but in detail there are a number of major differences.

In criminal cases the supreme court is the High Court of Justiciary which is based in Edinburgh but travels on circuit to many of the larger towns as well as the three other cities. The Lord Advocate or one of his Deputes always lead for the Crown, whilst the defence is in the hands of Advocates, not part of the Crown Office. Therefore the two forms of advocates are kept separate.

Lesser criminal matters are dealt with at the Sheriff Court. The Sheriff has jurisdiction over both criminal and civil matters and may sit in Summary Trials (without a jury) or in Solemn Procedure (with a jury of 15 persons). The prosecution is always in the hands of the Procurator Fiscal, or one of his several deputes.

The lowest court is the District Court, presided over by lay Justices (Magistrates) or by a Stipendiary Magistrate. The prosecution in these courts is again in the hands of the Procurator Fiscal, more often in those of one of his deputes. High Court Judges and Sheriffs are addressed as 'My Lord'; Justices are addressed as 'Your Honour'.

The highest civil court is the Court of Session, sitting in Edinburgh, but the majority of civil cases are heard in the Sheriff Courts. The highest court of appeal for civil cases is the House of Lords, whilst for criminal cases it is the Court of Criminal Appeal, in Edinburgh, unless there is a right of hearing for either jurisdiction in the European Court in Strasbourg.

Chapter 11
Drunkenness

Drunkenness is of medico-legal importance, partly because a drunken person is particularly liable to sustain injuries or to have accidents which may result in death or serious injury, and indeed he may die from the effects of the alcohol alone; and partly because the person may commit various offences while under the influence of alcohol.

Therefore at any time a doctor, whether in general practice or in a hospital department, may be required to examine a person suspected of being drunk. Where possible such an examination is better performed by a doctor accustomed to the procedure, such as a police surgeon, but this may not be possible, and so every doctor should have an elementary knowledge of how to make the examination. Otherwise not only is he liable to appear ridiculous when giving evidence in court, but he is liable to mistake some serious illness for drunkenness, with the result that the person will not receive appropriate treatment and may die.

Persons who are drunk may sustain serious injury or die because of:

1 Head injuries—e.g. extra or subdural haemorrhage following falls or fights. Not only will the drunken person be more aggressive or unsteady, but the presence of alcohol in the body makes bleeding more likely to occur, and in a chronic alcoholic the blood vessels may have become more fragile.

2 Falls from buildings, into areas or excavations, etc., may produce fractures, especially of the skull or neck.

3 Drowning—the drunken person may blunder into a river or canal. He may also collapse insensible in the street with his face in a puddle or gutter, and drown in a few inches of water.

4 Burns—by falls into fires or dropping cigarettes or lighted matches.

5 Electrocution—by fumbling with faulty apparatus.

6 Poisoning—formerly from carbon monoxide, by switching on the gas but forgetting to light it. By drinking other liquid poisons in mistake for water or further supplies of alcohol.

7 Asphyxia—from becoming trapped in confined spaces, becoming accidentally suspended, e.g. by clothing, smothering from bedclothes, strangulation from tight clothing during the alcoholic coma, or choking from the regurgitation and inhalation of stomach contents.

Drunkenness and the law

To be drunk is not an offence, unless the drunken person is behaving or performing some action to the annoyance or danger of other persons.

Drunken driving

Under the provisions of the Road Traffic Act 1988 it is an offence for a person to drive or attempt to drive a motor vehicle on a road or other public place if he is unfit to drive through drink or drugs; it is also an offence if he has an amount of alcohol in his blood greater than the prescribed limit, which is 80 mg of alcohol in 100 ml of blood (equivalent to 107 mg of alcohol in 100 ml of urine).

A police constable who suspects a motorist of having alcohol in his body or having committed a traffic offence can require him to take a breath test. The constable may then request the motorist to go to the police station in order to take a quantitative breath test, and if he refuses, may arrest him. At the police station the motorist will be required to take two breath tests on the quantitative instrument, the lower reading being the one used for evidence. If the reading of the machine is below the equivalent of 115 mg/100 ml of blood the motorist may choose to supply a confirmatory blood or urine sample. In some cases the motorist may be required to supply such a sample of blood or urine (Transport Act 1981).

In an endeavour to deal with problem drinking drivers, provision is made for all cases where the blood level exceeds 150 mg/100 ml to be notified to the Licensing Centre at Swansea. If a driver has two convictions within 10 years, the Licensing Centre will require evidence that his drink problem is under control before his licence is returned at the end of the usual period of disqualification. This will entail the driver attending at a special examination centre, where he will undergo medical examination, possibly including psychiatric examination.

Although refusal to supply any sample on the part of the driver is an offence, a police constable must obtain the permission of the medical officer in charge of the driver if he has been admitted to hospital; the medical officer can refuse permission if this would be prejudicial to the treatment of the patient.

The role of the doctor in this procedure is restricted to obtaining a blood sample with consent from the patient, and this responsibility usually devolves on the police surgeon. At the time when the sample is taken, in addition to the specimen handed to the police, part of the sample must be given to the motorist, in a sealed container, to enable him to obtain an independent analysis.

Drunk in various situations

Drunkenness may constitute an offence if on a passenger steamer, or in control of a child under 7 years, or in possession of loaded firearms, or in charge of horses or cattle, etc.

Overlaying of children

Under the Children and Young Persons Act 1933 any adult, over the age of 16, who, while under the influence of alcohol, takes a child under the age of 3 years into bed, as a result of which the child is suffocated by being overlayed, commits an offence.

In crimes of violence (e.g. murder)

Normally the fact that a person's mental attitude may be modified by alcohol, e.g. he may become more aggressive and so attack another, is not considered to reduce his responsibility for his actions. However it may be proved that at the time of the occurrence the accused was so hopelessly drunk as to be quite incapable of knowing what he was doing, or of forming any specific intention. This may reduce the offence from murder to manslaughter. Chronic alcoholism may amount to true insanity.

Physiology of alcohol

Alcohol is usually rapidly absorbed from the stomach, though this absorption may be slowed down if the stomach contains a meal, or especially fat, such as milk or olive oil. Most of a dose of alcohol will be absorbed from the stomach in 1 hour.

The alcohol then becomes distributed throughout the body, in proportion to the amount of water present in various tissues.

Elimination of the alcohol from the body is slower than its absorption. Most is metabolised, the average rate being 10 ml/hour, equal to a fall of 15 mg/100 ml/hour in the blood level of alcohol. There is considerable individual variation, however. About 90% of the ingested alcohol is removed in this way, the rest is excreted in the urine, breath and sweat.

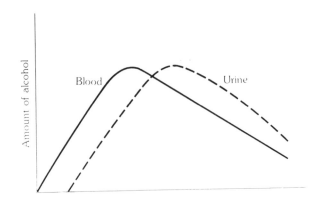

Ratio between blood and urine alcohol levels (Fig. 11.1)

During the time that alcohol is being absorbed the amount in the blood exceeds that in the urine. But once absorption ceases and elimination commences the level in the urine becomes greater than that in the blood at a given time in the ratio 4:3, since the urine obtained at a particular time is derived from blood passing through the kidneys some appreciable time before, when the blood level was higher. This is likely to apply at the time when the doctor makes his examination, and the known ratio makes it possible to calculate the level in the blood from an examination of the urine only. However, if there is any possibility of doubt then it is as well to take blood as well as urine samples.

Relation of blood alcohol level to symptoms

This will depend to a large extent on the person under examination, and how accustomed he is to taking alcohol, whether he is tired, or cold, or has taken any other drugs at the same time, or has disease such as cerebral arteriosclerosis.

0–50 mg/100 ml of blood: no symptoms likely.

50–150 mg/100 ml of blood: the levels usually reached during normal social drinking. The alcohol has produced some depression of higher centres and the person is talkative, and aggressive or friendly. The face and eyes are slightly suffused and there is a tendency to nystagmus, with dilated pupils.

150–250 mg/100 ml of blood: at this stage the person is intoxicated, as shown by muscular incoordination, slurred speech, impairment of memory, etc.

250–400 mg/100 ml of blood: the person at this level has reached the stage of pre-coma, is grossly uncoordinated with incoherent speech and sluggishly reacting pupils.

400–500 mg/100 ml of blood: the stage of coma has now been reached, with slow stertorous breathing, pallor, subnormal temperature and contracted pupils.

Over 500 mg/100 ml the high level of alcohol causes medullary paralysis, leading to death.

Examination of a suspected drunk

The amount of alcohol needed to be consumed to produce these levels varies greatly according to the size of the drinker, his stomach contents, etc. However, in very rough terms.

50 mg alcohol/100 ml blood = approximately 1½ pts beer
150 mg   ”   ”   ”   =   ”   4 pts beer
250 mg   ”   ”   ”   =   ”   7 pts beer
400 mg   ”   ”   ”   =   ”   11 pts beer

The ability to decide whether a person is under the influence of alcohol, or whether he is suffering from some disease or injury is a matter of clinical judgement, only acquired by practice. Therefore, where possible, it is better for such examinations to be conducted by doctors with special experience, e.g. police surgeons. Since, under the provisions of the Road Traffic Act 1972, most prosecutions are likely to be based on the results of analysis of blood or urine samples, clinical examinations to assess drunkenness are much less frequently required than formerly. However, in special circumstances a doctor may be required to make such an examination. The following notes only give the very general outline of the procedure. For greater detail the student should consult the BMA pamphlet, *The Recognition of Intoxication* (1954).

Time of examination

If requested to make the examination the doctor should attend as quickly as possible, since the effects of intoxication may begin to wear off, and if the patient is suffering from some other condition he may be in danger. The time when the doctor is called, and when he begins his examination should be recorded.

Consent to examination

Before making any examination the doctor should obtain the consent of the patient, in writing and witnessed. He must explain the nature and the purpose of the examination he proposes to make and that his findings will be made known to the police. He must also explain what samples he proposes to take.

The doctor must at this stage make it clear that the patient is not obliged to submit to an examination, and that he is entitled to insist that the examination is conducted by a doctor of his own choice.

If the patient is incapable of giving consent by reason of unconsciousness or gross intoxication, then the doctor may make an examination, take samples, and give such treatment as is necessary to save life. However, he may not divulge the results of his examination until he can obtain the consent of the patient, or the patient dies, except when directed to do so by a court.

Purpose of examination

The aim of the doctor should be to decide whether the patient is under the influence of alcohol, and if so to what extent, e.g. is his ability to drive properly impaired; or is his condition due to illness or injury; or is it safe for him to be detained in a police station, or should he be admitted to hospital.

Form of examination

(As given in the BMA pamphlet.)

1   The presence of any serious injury or acute illness requiring immediate attention should be excluded at once.

2   History, e.g. of previous illness, fits, etc., of the nature of any recent food or drink, and whether the patient is taking any drugs.

3   General behaviour—state of dress, speech and self-control.

4   Memory and mental state—questions of name and address, date and time, and simple arithmetic.

5   Writing—copying from book or newspaper.

6   Pulse—temperature, skin condition.

7   Mouth—state of tongue, nature of teeth, smell of breath.

8   Eyes—general appearance, glass eyes, pupil reactions, eye movements.

9   Ears—impairment of hearing, condition of drums.

10   Gait—on walking across a room and turning (not along a straight line).

11   Stance—with eyes open and closed.

12   Coordination—finger-nose test, picking up objects, performing simple acts such as buttoning clothing.

13   Reflexes and general CNS examination.

14   Examinations of cardiovascular, respiratory, and alimentary systems.

Diagnosis

This must be based on the whole of the results of the examination, not on isolated features such as the smell of the breath.

The doctor's report to the police must only deal with matters for which he was asked to make the examination, e.g. the presence of intoxication, the presence of other disease, and the fitness of the person to be detained. These opinions must only relate to the patient at the time of the examination. No opinion should be given of the patient's condition at some time earlier than the examination.

Specimens

These usually consist of urine or breath samples, and arrangements for obtaining these will have been made by the police, so that the doctor is not concerned. Blood samples may be requested by the police or by the patient, and can only be taken with the consent of the patient. The sample must be divided into two, one part being given to the police, the other to the patient. The object is to allow the person to obtain an independent analysis if he wishes. Alcohol must not be used to sterilise the skin or the syringe, of course.

The patient may refuse to allow a sample to be taken, but this may be taken by the court subsequently to support the prosecution's case, or may constitute an offence under the provisions of the Road Traffic Act 1988.

'Special' kits containing receptacles for the blood, etc., are held by the police. The receptacles must contain fluoride to prevent enzymatic decomposition of the blood. After filling they must be kept cool, but not frozen or heated. Once in the sealed container, the seal must not be broken until the sample reaches the analyst.

Chapter 12
Sexual Offences

Types of offence

These are set out in the Sexual Offences Act 1956, as amended by the Sexual Offences Act 1967, in respect of homosexual acts and the Sexual Offences (Amendments) Act 1976.

In **Scotland** most of the offences are defined at common law, but one statute is the Sexual Offences (Scotland) Act 1976. In Northern Ireland the Homosexual Offences (Northern Ireland) Order 1982 has brought the law there more closely into line with English practice.

Rape

This is defined, in the 1976 Act, as unlawful sexual intercourse with a woman without her consent, the man knowing that she does not consent, or is reckless whether she consents or not.

Note

1 Sexual intercourse, within the meaning of the Act, is constituted by any degree of penetration from mere entry of the tip of the penis between the labia majora to full penetration into the vagina, with or without emission of seminal fluid. The point is that conception may occur without full penetration, if semen is deposited at the vulva, and moreover, the degree of emotional shock may be equally great whether or not full penetration has occurred.

2 Sexual intercourse with an adult woman may be lawful, if she gives consent, and is always lawful in marriage unless the parties are legally separated, the marriage contract implying consent of the wife to intercourse. Therefore a man cannot rape his wife, though his conduct may constitute cruelty, sufficient to justify divorce, or the offences of wounding or assault, or causing grievous bodily harm.

3 'By force and against her will' includes not only the actual use of bodily violence to restrain or coerce the woman, but also the threat of violence, and also includes the use of drugs to stupefy the woman, and the use of fraud such as impersonation of the husband.

Intercourse with children

Intercourse with girls under the age of 16 years is always illegal, even if consent is given; such consent is always invalid. However, girls who are close to

16 years of age may dress and behave as though they were much older, and deceive the unwary male. Therefore the law creates two classes of offence.
1   Intercourse with a girl under 13 years of age. This is considered a grave offence, ranking with rape.
2   Intercourse with a girl between 13 and 16 years of age, unless accomplished by force and against her will, in which case it will be rape, is a less grave offence, punishable with up to 2 years' imprisonment.

There may be a valid defence to a charge of the latter offence, if it is shown that the accused man was under 24 years, he genuinely believed and had reasonable cause to believe that the girl was over 16 years old, and he had never before been *charged* with a like offence.

Intercourse with mental defectives

It is an offence, punishable by 2 years' imprisonment, for a man to have intercourse with a woman who is suffering from mental subnormality or severe subnormality, or a patient under the care of a mental hospital, or under guardianship unless it can be shown that the man was not aware of the mental state of the woman.

Incest

It is an offence for a man to have intercourse with his granddaughter, daughter, sister, half-sister or mother. Similarly a woman may not have intercourse with her grandson, son, brother, half-brother or father.

If intercourse is with a girl under 13 years of age, then as before, this is a grave offence punishable by life imprisonment, otherwise punishment may be up to 7 years' imprisonment.

Indecent assault

This offence can be committed by either a man or a woman. Indeed a woman cannot be charged with the rape of a man or boy, but can be charged with indecent assault.

The range of acts constituting such an assault is wide, from handling the genitalia to merely disarranging the clothing.

As in the case of sexual intercourse, an adult woman can give consent to such behaviour, as in courtship, and in that case no offence is committed. However, girls under the age of 16 years, and mental defectives, cannot give valid consent for such behaviour, which in their case, therefore, always constitutes an offence.

Because the range of acts constituting such an offence is so wide, any persons who have to examine or interview members of the opposite sex such as doctors are always at risk from false or mistaken allegations of misconduct, unless the utmost care is taken with regard to chaperons, etc. Doctors and dentists are particularly at risk when administering anaesthetics to female patients, since erotic dreams, followed by discovery of disordered clothing on recovering consciousness, may lead to the genuinely mistaken belief on the patient's part that she has been assaulted.

Examination of an alleged victim of sexual offence

Before conducting such an examination, remember:

1   An allegation of rape may be false. Such allegations may be from spite, jealousy, in order to precipitate marriage, etc.

2   The doctor must endeavour to show whether or not sexual intercourse has taken place, and to note any injuries. He cannot say whether rape has occurred. Penetration and emission of semen with bruises and teeth marks may occur in consenting intercourse. Equally, a rape can occur without full penetration or emission and without the production of any injuries.

3   The offence is a grave charge, so if possible, examination should only be performed by a doctor having special experience of such cases.

Scheme of examination

Consent

Obtain written consent from the girl, or her parent or guardian if she is under 16 years.

Premises

Ensure that the examination can be conducted in suitable premises, such as the doctor's surgery; not in some ill-lit waiting-room of a police station.

History

Take a history of the occurrence, if possible, both from the girl and separately from some other person in whom she has confided, e.g. the mother. Note both the date and time of the examination, and also the date and time of the alleged incident.

It is important to know, for instance;

1   The place of the incident; house, wood, etc.
2   The course of events during the incident.
3   The relative position of the parties.
4   The steps taken by the victim to resist.
5   Whether the victim lost consciousness at any time.
6   Whether she was menstruating at the time.

General appearance

While taking the history, note the general appearance and behaviour of the girl, signs of distress or discomfort, apparent age and physique, and whether she dresses or looks older than her age.

Clothing

Enquire whether the clothing worn at the examination is that worn when the attack occurred. If so, it should be examined for damage, tears, stains, etc., and arrangements made for it to be sent to a forensic science laboratory for examination, ensuring that it is safely packed to avoid contamination, in polythene or brown paper bags provided by the police, and labelled, with the doctor's initials or identifying mark on the label to allow identification subsequently in court.

Physical examination

General. It is important to examine the whole of the body for injuries, notably bruises and abrasions, especially on the thighs, from separating the legs, on the arms from gripping, on the back of the shoulders from forcibly holding down, and on the face and neck from prevention of the woman crying out. Also bite or suction marks, oval bruises, may be found on the neck or on the breasts, and the nipples may be bitten. Note her physique, in relation to the amount of resistance of which she would be capable.

Of the genitalia. This follows the pattern of a normal gynaecological examination, but especially noting:
1 Pubic hair. Any matting by semen. Remember to take a sample, but not until the end of the examination, since the hairs should be plucked, not cut.
2 Vulva. Look for swelling, reddening, abrasions, lacerations, and tenderness.
3 Hymen. Look for a fresh tear of the hymen, with reddening and tenderness of the margins. Old tears are of no assistance, and in a married woman the hymen may be absent. Even in a virgin it may be so elastic as to be undamaged by intercourse, particularly if tampons have been regularly used.
4 Vagina. Look for bruising, abrasion, or laceration of the walls. Dilatation of the vagina is not necessarily proof of intercourse, it may be due to the use of tampons or masturbation. A sample of vaginal fluid should be taken for examination for spermatozoa. The sample may be taken either by capillary pipette, and smears prepared on microscope slides, or by means of a damp throat swab. In either case, if the sample has to be sent any distance to the laboratory, smears should be prepared at once, and allowed to dry on the slides, otherwise the sperms will disintegrate.

The swabs should be sent as well as the smears, however, so that bacteriological examination can be made for venereal disease, and if this is thought possible it would be as well for the swabs to be sent in some transport medium.

Any fibres or foreign hairs found on the genitalia should be preserved and sent for examination, as well as a sample of the girl's pubic hair, and also a blood sample for grouping.

Note that the object of the examination is (a) to determine whether intercourse has taken place, by finding seminal fluid in the vagina, and (b) to note any injuries to the body or genitalia denoting forceful intercourse, or a struggle, but remembering that such injuries do not necessarily indicate rape.

Examination of a person accused of rape

It is unlikely a doctor will be called upon to make such an examination unless he is a police surgeon or prison medical officer. However, the general principles of such an examination are as follows:

1 *Obtain written consent* for the examination, after explaining its purpose.

2 Take a history of the circumstances of the intercourse. The man's story can then be compared with the girl's and with the facts of the examination.

3 Note any stains on the clothing. Their identification is a job for the forensic science laboratory.

4 Note the man's age and physique. Look for injuries which might have been sustained during a struggle, such as nail scratches on the face.

5 Note the size of the penis, and look for injuries to it, such as a tear of the frenum. Look for evidence of active venereal disease.

6 Take samples of pubic hair, and also blood samples for grouping.

Seminal fluid

Possible seminal staining of clothes may be indicated by fluorescence under ultraviolet light, but many other substances can also fluoresce. Seminal fluid contains the enzyme acid phosphatase, and so tests for this enzyme on suspected stains or fluid will be made in the laboratory. However, the most reliable proof is the demonstration of intact spermatozoa. Seminal fluid, in a person who is a secreter, will contain blood group substances, and can be grouped by the ABO and PGM systems, and by DNA profiling.

Anal intercourse

Sexual intercourse per anum has always been regarded as unnatural, and a crime of considerable gravity, a felony known as buggery. It was immaterial whether the act was performed on a man or a woman. However, the Sexual Offences Act 1967, recognising the existence and needs of homosexual persons, has made the act lawful as between consenting adults, performing in private. (A public lavatory is specifically excluded as a private place.)

It is still unlawful for the act to be performed on a person who does not give consent, including those, i.e. children, who cannot give consent. The age at which a person becomes an adult for the purposes of this Act is 21 years. (A boy under 14 is sexually immature and cannot be accused of rape, or buggery. He can be accused of indecent assault.)

Therefore, the doctor may be called upon to examine a person who alleges anal intercourse has been practised on him without consent, and also possibly the person who is alleged to have performed the act.

Medical examination

The passive agent. If seen soon after an act of anal intercourse, performed for the first time, the anal wall may be painful, reddened, grazed and bruised. There may be small fresh tears of the wall. There may be traces of lubricant in the anal canal, such as petroleum jelly, and also seminal fluid, which must be retained for examination on slides or a swab as in the case of rape.

Where anal intercourse is frequently practised, the anal canal becomes dilated and its wall scarred, due to old tears. It will tend to dilate when the buttocks are separated. There may be evidence of venereal disease. The doctor must beware of mistaking natural disease, such as anal fissure or rectal prolapse, for evidence of anal intercourse.

The active agent. Little is likely to be found here, except for possibly fresh injury to the penis and traces of faecal material on the glans.

Bestiality

This is sexual intercourse with animals, a form of sexual perversion obviously more likely to be encountered in the country. Proof is usually a matter of investigation by the police and by forensic scientists, and the doctor is not likely to be involved.

Part 2
Forensic Pathology

Chapter 13
Examination of the Dead

The first and principal duty of a doctor who is called to the scene of a death is to ascertain that death has in fact occurred. Lack of care in this examination has caused some embarrassing moments when 'bodies' have revived in the mortuary, notably of persons suffering from hypothermia, electrocution or poisoning. If the person is still alive, or the fact of death is not certain after examination, the doctor's only concern should be the welfare of the patient.

Two types of death are described, somatic death which is extinction of personality when vital processes cease, and molecular death, when the tissues of the body begin to disintegrate. The diagnosis of somatic death is of greater practical importance, and with modern apparatus for transfusion, artificial respiration, cardiac stimulation, etc., it may be difficult to decide at what moment a person has ceased to be an individual, and has become a mass of tissues being artificially maintained by the therapeutic procedures.

Signs of death

Death is considered to have occurred when the vital functions, e.g. breathing and heart beat, have irreversibly ceased. In hospital this may if necessary be firmly established by the use of investigations such as ECG (electrocardiogram) or EEG (electroencephalograph). Otherwise the absence of any heart or breath sounds on auscultation over a period of 5 minutes is sufficient indication. Other old-fashioned tests such as mirrors or feathers on the mouth or ligatures around the finger are quite unreliable.

Examination of the eye with an ophthalmoscope may confirm the cessation of the circulation by showing breaking up of the columns of blood in the retinal blood vessels.

If there is any doubt, e.g. dubious heart sounds heard during an examination in a noisy street, it is obviously safer to assume that the person is still alive and send him at once to hospital where EEG or even auscultation in quiet surroundings may settle the issue.

Associated with the failure of vital functions are the pallor of the skin, flaccidity of muscles and dilated pupils which make up the 'dead' appearance, but which are too imprecise to serve as criteria for the diagnosis of death.

Deciding when a patient is dead may present particular difficulties if respiration and circulation are being maintained artificially by a respirator.

The usual criteria cannot then be applied and instead a diagnosis of 'brain death' has to be made.

The procedure for establishing this has been described in a statement issued by the Royal Colleges. In summary, the patient must be deeply comatose, maintained on a ventilator because of lack of spontaneous respiration, and suffering from irremediable structural brain damage, of known cause. Brain death is confirmed by the absence of all brain-stem reflexes; for instance the corneal, vestibulo-ocular, and gag reflexes and the absence of respiratory movements when the respirator is disconnected. Other investigations, such as EEG and cerebral angiography may be used, but are not necessary to establish the diagnosis.

Bodily changes after death

Some of the earlier of these changes, such as cooling of the body, and rigor mortis, are confirmatory evidence that death has occurred. All of them are of value in indicating approximately when death occurred.

Cooling

Theoretically this starts as soon as life ceases, and continues for about 18–24 hours, until the body temperature reaches that of its surroundings, at an average rate of 1.5°F (0.9°C)/hour. The actual rate may vary between about 3°F (1.8°C) and 0.5°F (0.3°C)/hour, depending on whether death has only recently occurred, or took place many hours previously, i.e. the difference in temperature between the body and its surroundings is great or little. The rate of fall will also be slowed in a well-clothed body or one which is fat, and hastened in a naked or thin body, or one immersed in water.

To obtain a rough approximation of the time of death, from the extent of cooling, divide the number of degrees of temperature lost from 99°F (37°C) by 1.5 (i.e. allowing for a rate of cooling of 1.5°F or 0.9°C/hour). But it must be remembered that this is only an approximation; the body may not commence to cool for several hours after death, or the temperature at or soon after death may exceed the normal 98.4°F (37°C) by up to 7°F (4.2°C). Therefore these factors can introduce an error of several hours in the estimated time of death. The temperature must be recorded in the rectum, not on the body surface, using a long chemical thermometer, or a low-reading variety. Electric thermo-couples are being increasingly used nowadays and some experts have produced nomograms, enabling the time of death to be read off a chart.

Hypostasis

After death blood drains in the relaxed and dilated vessels by gravity to the lowest parts of the body. This process starts at death, but is not normally apparent for 4–6 hours, and is fully established in about 12 hours. After 12 hours the blood becomes coagulated in the vessels, so that if a body is rolled over after this time the hypostasis will not alter its distribution, and will be seen on the uppermost part of the body. The hypostasis is often difficult to see in a fat person or one who has lost much blood recently. Its colour may indicate chemical changes in the blood during life, e.g. pink due to carboxyhaemoglobin or grey-brown due to methaemoglobin.

Rigor mortis

This stiffening of the muscles is due to gelling of muscle protein, due to exhaustion of glycolysis and metabolism of ATP. It affects the smaller muscles of the jaw and the extremities before the larger muscle masses. Under normal conditions the stiffening will be apparent in about 6 hours, and will have affected the whole body in 12 hours. This stiffness of the body will last for about 36–48 hours, before passing off as putrefaction begins to dissolve the muscle protein. This time pattern is, however, subject to considerable variation. A person who has been using his muscles violently, e.g. in fight or flight, will have an accumulation of the products of glucose metabolism already present in the muscles at death, and so rigor will develop more rapidly. For the same reasons certain poisons such as strychnine will hasten the onset of rigor. On the other hand slow lingering deaths, where the muscle supplies of glucose are depleted, will be associated with slower and weaker development of rigor. Also the rate at which rigor passes off will obviously be related to the speed of onset of putrefaction, which may be very rapid in hot environments.

Once a stiffened muscle, in rigor, is stretched, and the rigor 'broken' stiffening will not recur.

Other causes of stiffening of muscles:

1   In extensive burns, where the heat 'cooks' the muscle protein.

2   In intense cold when the joints are frozen; on thawing the muscles will pass into rigor.

3   Cadaveric spasm; a rare condition of unknown mechanism, in which in sudden violent deaths, groups of muscles or the whole body may suddenly stiffen at the moment of death, e.g. the hand holding a weapon used in a suicidal attempt.

Putrefaction

The presence of this process is not likely to be in doubt, when fully developed. Its early stages consist of a greenish discoloration of the skin of the anterior abdominal wall over the right iliac fossa, soon spreading to the whole of the abdominal wall, appearing at about 48 hours after death in normal conditions. Subsequently the body swells and discoloration appears along the lines of the superficial veins (marbling), with blistering of the skin, rupture of body cavities and liquefaction of organs.

The temperature of the environment will of course affect the speed of onset of the putrefaction.

Adipocere

This change does not usually become apparent for some months after death. It consists of a hydrolysis of body fats to fatty acids and soaps, the end product, adipocere, being a white greasy musty-smelling material, which by replacing the fatty tissue, may maintain the outline of the part or even the whole of the body. It is most commonly found in bodies lying in relatively warm moist anaerobic situations, e.g. clothed bodies buried in poorly-drained soil. If the soil is very acid, e.g. peat bog, an alternative process akin to tanning may preserve the entire body in an excellent state, as in certain archaeological discoveries, notably in Denmark, and recently in the United Kingdom (Lindow Man).

In warm, dry environments, the body may become dry and brittle, and dark brown in colour, the process being known as mummification.

Post-mortem mutilation

After death a body may be exposed to the attacks of animals and insects. The animals, either domestic, such as cats, or wild as rats or foxes, may cause severe damage, during the first few days after death, which can be distinguished from injuries caused in life by the presence of minute scratches or toothmarks at the margins of the injuries. The onset of putrefaction may be accompanied by infestation by maggots or beetle larvae. The species present, or the stage of their development may indicate to an entymologist the approximate period that has elapsed since death.

Estimating the time of death—survey

Death
0–12 hours	Body temperature
24 hours	Rigor mortis and hypostasis
48 hours–3 weeks	Putrefaction
Months–years	Adipocere and mummification

Visiting the scene of death

This is likely to occur in one of two circumstances:

1 On a routine visit to see the body of a dead patient before the doctor issues a death certificate, where there are no suspicious circumstances.

2 Visiting the scene of a death in suspicious circumstances, summoned by the police.

Circumstances not suspicious

Obviously such cases are almost always ordinary deaths from natural causes, and to treat each one in a manner that implied to the relatives that one suspected foul play would be ridiculous. However unless the doctor was actually present at the moment of death, he should always have suspicions, though keeping them to himself. Thus having confirmed the fact of death he should check the body to eliminate the presence of any injuries, examining especially the neck, and the back of the body. He should note any tablets or cups in the room or by the bed, which might indicate that poison had been taken, and should see if the deceased had left any notes. He should not omit to ask any relatives or neighbours for details of the death, and if he is in doubt about the cause of death, he should inform the Coroner or Procurator Fiscal. Common causes of sudden unexpected death are myocardial ischaemia due to coronary atheroma or coronary thrombosis, pulmonary embolism due to leg vein thrombosis, cerebral haemorrhage due to aneurysm or hypertension, and ruptured abdominal aneurysms. Severe infections such as pneumonia or peritonitis may develop rapidly and be unsuspected, especially in elderly persons living on their own. However, the likelihood of a natural cause for sudden death must not blind the doctor to the presence of carbon monoxide poisoning, or a fractured femur.

Suspicious circumstances

In such circumstances the doctor will usually be asked to attend by the police, who are probably treating the case as one of murder until it has been confirmed, or proved otherwise. The principal things for the doctor to bear in mind are:

1   To enquire what is required of him, i.e. is he simply required to establish the fact of death, or to make a more detailed examination.

2   To be sure not to go beyond the scope of his competency, i.e. not to be afraid to admit if he is unfamiliar with the particular type of death.

3   To be careful not to interfere with the investigations of others, i.e. by destroying fingerprints, stains, suicide notes, etc.

It is obviously important to attend at the scene of death as quickly as possible. On arrival the doctor should obtain a brief statement of the circumstances, and enquire what is required of him. He should also enquire what he must not touch, the golden rule being to touch as little as possible and to displace nothing.

His most important function is to ascertain that death has occurred, with as little disturbance as possible. However, if he thinks that life is still present, or he cannot be sure, then all other things must be subordinated to the treatment of the person. If death had undoubtedly occurred, he should try to form an opinion as to the approximate time of death from the state of rigor, hypostasis, etc. Any interference with the body, such as to record the body temperature, should only be with the agreement of the police officers, lest important evidence is disturbed. He should check that the identity of the deceased is correct, and he should endeavour to ascertain the cause of death, from the presence of obvious marks or injuries such as the mark of a ligature on the neck. He should note the position and state of clothing of the body before it is moved, and make a quick sketch plan to refresh his memory later and he should make a note of such things as the type and distribution of any bloodstains, cups, tablets, weapons, etc., in the area.

These things should be recorded in writing as soon as possible, preferably at the scene, with the time of the investigation, the names of the relevant police officers, the address of the premises, etc., so that if the case comes to court in 2 to 3 months' time the doctor can refresh his memory, from his original notes. He should remember that although at the time he may apparently not be required to do much, and may appear to have a very minor role, months later his recollection and observation of facts may figure largely in court proceedings, if only to corroborate or refute others' evidence.

Medico-legal autopsy

It is very unlikely that a general practitioner would be called upon to perform a medico-legal autopsy, therefore it is not proposed to make any detailed description of the methods employed. Such an examination should only be performed by a pathologist having special experience in this field. Details of who may be called upon to perform such autopsies, and of the type of examination required are contained in the Coroners Rules (1953) or the Rules for Procurators Fiscal (1985). The principles of the examination are:

1   To make precise records of when and where the autopsy was performed, and in whose presence.

2   To remember the possible hazards of infections such as AIDS or hepatitis B if the deceased was a suspected drug addict or promiscuous homosexual.

3   To remember to examine the clothing.

4   To make a detailed and meticulous external examination of the body, noting especially any marks on the neck, the hands, and the genitalia, and remembering to examine the back of the body and the scalp.

5   To enquire at this stage whether any samples are required by the police, such as specimens of hair or/and nail scrapings, and to give the police opportunity to take photographs, finger-prints, etc.

6   During the internal examination to remember to open all the body cavities, including the skull, to measure the amounts of blood or other fluids present in the cavities, to trace the direction and depth of injuries before the organs are removed, and to measure and record all injuries found however trivial they may appear.

7 To remember to retain the gastric contents and samples of blood and urine while this is possible.

8 To ensure that all the samples are kept separately in clean glass containers, are labelled in a way that will enable the doctor to identify them months later, and are handed to the appropriate police officer, whose name the doctor will record.

9 To retain tissues or organs which have a bearing on the death, e.g. any wound, or neck structures in cases of strangulation, preserved in a way that will make them of use to any other doctor requiring to see them, e.g. a pathologist acting on behalf of the defence.

Autopsy report

The report on a medico-legal autopsy follows the same general pattern as any autopsy report, e.g. details of the deceased, external findings, internal findings arranged by systems, and conclusions as to cause of death. The precise form varies from one pathologist to another.

However in medico-legal cases it is important to remember the following:

1 The report is the property of the Coroner or Procurator Fiscal, and copies may not be given to anyone else without his permission.

2 So far as is possible, consistent with accuracy, the report should be in simple language, avoiding technical terms, since it will have to be read and understood by various layman at different stages of the investigation.

Chapter 14
Blood

Bloodstains

At the scene of a death the doctor's main duty is to examine the body. Other experts, forensic scientists, fingerprint specialists, police photographers, etc., will be responsible for examining the surroundings, and the doctor must be very careful to avoid inadvertently destroying valuable evidence by handling or moving objects.

However, the interpretation of the nature and distribution of bloodstains, in an attempt to determine the circumstances of the death, may be expected of the doctor, either at the scene, or later, in court.

The different kinds of bloodstains which may be present can be considered under three headings:
1 Blood on and around the body.
2 Blood spots and splashes on walls, furniture, etc.
3 Smears, or trails of blood on floors.

Blood on and around the body

Almost any dead body bearing wounds is likely to be lying in a pool of blood, part of which has probably drained out after death. The absence of such a pool is more noteworthy as it suggests that the body has been moved after death. The amount of blood present in relation to the size of the injury is deceptive; a minor injury such as a ruptured varicose vein or a laceration of an eyebrow may produce a large pool of blood, compared to a much more deeply penetrating stab-wound which may have pierced the aorta but where most of the bleeding is into the body cavities.

It may be useful to note the position of bloodstains on the body particularly the linear stains produced by blood running across the body from the wound. For instance, signs of blood having trickled down the legs of a body which is found lying on the floor, with a stab-wound in the chest, indicates that the deceased was upright when the wound was inflicted.

Blood spots and spashes on walls, furniture, etc.

These spots may have been produced by blood dripping from a wounded person who was staggering around the room, from spurts of blood escaping from a severed artery, or as spray from a bloodstained weapon wielded by an assailant. This may be determined from the position and shape of the spots; a line of blood spots on the ceiling are likely to have come from a

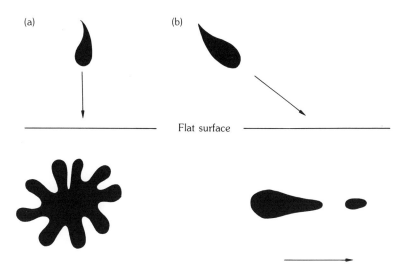

Fig. 14.1. Shape of blood drops. (a) Drop landing vertically; (b) drop landing obliquely.

bloodstained weapon; rounded spots on the floor or flat surfaces of furniture probably were produced by blood dripping from the victim.

The direction is which the blood was travelling, and hence the likely point from which it originated, can be determined from the shape of the blood spots. Thus blood dropping vertically on to a flat surface makes a rounded spot which may have a crenated margin if the spot has travelled for some distance. A drop arriving obliquely at the surface will produce a splash in the shape of an exclamation mark, the smaller spot pointing the direction in which the blood was travelling (Fig. 14.1).

Smears and trails of blood on floors

These are produced when the person crawls, or his body is dragged, after wounding. They may consist of a series of drops of blood, or of blood smears on the floor, doorposts, etc. The smears will tend to become indistinct and have a ragged margin in the direction of travel (Fig. 14.2).

Apart from noting and interpreting the position of such bloodstains the doctor may have an important function in ensuring that they are preserved until they can be photographed, by pointing them out to the investigating police officers, or by preventing relatives or bystanders from disturbing the scene of death until the police arrive.

Laboratory examination of bloodstains

This is obviously a specialist's field, and a detailed knowledge of the various methods used is never likely to be required by the average doctor. Therefore the following account is only a brief outline of the procedure, designed to

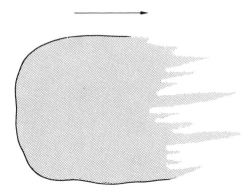

Fig. 14.2. Shape of blood smear.

indicate the scope of the investigations, and the purpose of preserving samples.

Summary (Fig. 14.3)

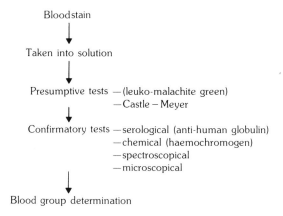

Fig. 14.3. Summary of laboratory procedure for examining bloodstains.

Preparation of solution

Before most of the tests can be applied the stain must be taken into solution, by soaking the stained fabric, or fragments of the dried stain scraped from the surface of a weapon or piece of furniture, in normal saline.

Presumptive tests

There are several of these, designed to distinguish stains made by blood or other body fluids from those made by paint, rust, fruit juice, etc.

Most laboratories now use the leuko-malachite green test, in which a solution of the reagent is added to the stain, followed by hydrogen peroxide. A blue-green colour results with blood. The Castle–Meyer test (reduced phenolphthalein) is also used.

These tests are useful as screening procedures, to determine which stains deserve further investigation, and also to detect minute traces of blood at a scene, in a washbasin for instance. A filter-paper may be rubbed on the stain, and the test then applied to the filter-paper.

Confirmatory tests

1   *Serological.* These methods are the most commonly used of the various confirmatory procedures, having the merits of speed and specificity. Precipitin tests with anti-human globulin, or other antisera, will confirm that the substance causing the stain is blood, and will indicate whether the blood is human, or animal.

2   *Chemical.* There are several different tests. Reagents are used to produce derivatives of haemoglobin which have characteristic crystalline forms, visible by microscopic examination. A well-known example of such a method is Takayama's haemochromogen test.

3   *Spectroscopic.* A solution of reduced haemoglobin has a characteristic absorption spectrum. The test is made more specific by adding various reagents to the solution of the stain, to produce different products of haemoglobin, such as methaemoglobin, which have their own characteristic spectrum.

4   *Microscopical.* In a dried bloodstain the various formed elements of the blood, red and white cells, etc., are usually destroyed. However, red cells can occasionally be identified, if the stain is reasonably fresh, and their appearance may allow the source of the blood to be identified. Thus the red cells of avian blood are nucleated, and those from a camel are oval (information which is fascinating, but rarely of practical value).

Grouping of bloodstains

Various techniques have been developed by forensic scientists, which depend basically on the absorption by the stain of the specific antibodies from test solutions. The absorbed antibodies are then eluted from the stain, and their presence indicated by agglutination of fresh red cells of known groups.

Thus a dried stain of group B blood will absorb anti-B agglutinins, but not anti-A. The absorbed agglutinins can then be eluted, and will agglutinate known group B red cells.

Such tests can be performed on solutions of the stains, or even on a few fibres from the stained fabric.

The extent of blood group determination usually includes the ABO system and polymorphic enzyme groups, such as PGM. It is restricted by the condition of the stains and the amount of material available. For the same reason the application of the new technique of DNA profiling is of limited value, being more often applied to samples of seminal fluid.

It should be remembered that other body fluids, such as saliva or semen, may contain blood group substances, and can be grouped in the same way. About 70% of the population, known as secretors, have such blood group substance in their body fluids.

Blood samples

From living persons

Such samples are usually required from persons accused of drunken driving, or persons accused of assault or murder. It is important for the doctor who is asked to take such samples to remember:

1 To ensure that the person from whom the sample is to be taken understands the nature of the procedure, and the purpose for which the sample is required, and gives valid consent, in writing.

2 Not to sterilise the skin with alcohol if the sample is later to be analysed for alcohol.

3 To ensure in the case of a 'drunken driver' that the sample is divided into two parts, one to be handed to the police for analysis and one to be given to the accused person so that he may have an independent analysis performed if he wishes.

4 To see that the samples are securely labelled, in a manner that will enable the doctor to identify them later in court.

5 To make a note of whom he hands the labelled samples to, e.g. the name of the police officer, in case the doctor is asked this in court, when continuity of evidence is being established.

6 The possible hazards of infection by AIDS or hepatitis B should be remembered if taking blood samples from someone who is a known, or suspected, drug addict or promiscuous homosexual.

At autopsy

Such samples are required either for determination of the deceased's blood group, to compare with the groups of bloodstains on weapons or clothing, or for analysis for alcohol or poisons.

The principles for taking blood samples in the living as regards labelling also apply here. In addition the site from which the blood sample is taken may be important. For grouping purposes it is not necessary that the blood come from any particular site, i.e. it can be taken from the heart or from a peripheral vein, but when taking samples for alcohol estimation the blood should only be taken from a peripheral vein, if possible the femoral vein, to avoid the confusion which may arise from the post-mortem changes in alcohol content, which may occur in the blood in the vicinity of the liver. If other poisons are suspected samples of blood from the heart and from peripheral veins should be collected separately, since the variation in the amount of drug in different parts of the circulation may assist in determining how much of the poison was taken, and at what length of time before death. Blood samples should never be scooped up from blood lying free in body cavities unless there is absolutely no other source available. If this has to be done, the analyst must be informed of the source of the blood.

If the blood is not to be taken at once to the laboratory, it should be kept in a refrigerator at about 4°C if possible, and a small amount of sodium fluoride added to prevent enzymatic decomposition of alcohol.

As regards the amount of the sample, the more that can be obtained the better, but even very small samples may be valuable, since modern methods for the analysis of alcohol, CO, etc., and for blood grouping require only very small amounts.

Chapter 15
Wounds

Laws of wounding

Offences Against the Person Act 1861 (not applicable to Scotland)

The offences named range from assault, even if only by a threatening gesture, and battery, when a blow is struck, to causing actual bodily harm, or grievous bodily harm, or unlawful wounding, and to manslaughter or murder when the victim dies as a result of the injury. Thus a doctor may find himself required to examine a living person with an injury, or the body of a person who has died from wounds.

The difference between murder and manslaughter is one of intent. Wounding a person with intent to kill or cause grievous bodily harm so that he dies, constitutes murder. Wounding a person so as to cause his or her death without such intent, e.g. during a brawl or chastisement, would constitute manslaughter. In Scotland, wounding or injuring as the result of an assault, is not spelled-out in any specific statute. They are injuries at common law. Whereas murder in England is defined as the unlawful killing of a person with malice aforethought, being either express or implied and resulting in death within a year and a day, in Scotland, murder is simply an intentionally committed homicide and is not time barred. In England an unintentional killing is defined as manslaughter; the term in Scotland is culpable homicide, but the distinction between it and murder is not clearly delineated.

Homicide Act 1957 (not applicable to Scotland)

This divided the crime of murder into two categories, capital murder, for which the punishment was death, and non-capital murder, punishable by imprisonment. At that time capital murder comprised murder during the course of theft, by shooting, and of police or prison officers while resisting arrest. Subsequently (in 1965) the death penalty was abolished.

The Act also made provision for the defence of diminished responsibility, where a person who killed another would not be convicted of murder if at the time he suffered from an abnormality of mind so as to substantially impair his mental responsibility for his acts.

Suicide Act 1961

By this Act a person who commits or attempts to commit suicide is no longer guilty of any crime. On the other hand a person who assists another to commit suicide, such as the surviving partner of a suicide pact, is guilty of manslaughter.

External injuries

Bruises

These are the result of blows with blunt objects rupturing small blood vessels, with bleeding into the adjacent tissues. The bleeding may continue for some time after the blow has been struck, and it is likely to be greater in amount in children, old people, women and anyone suffering from deficiency diseases or haematological disorders. Therefore the size of the bruise is unreliable as an indication of the amount of force causing it. Moreover, although the striking object will have had a shape, this will not be reproduced by the bruise because the continued bleeding will blur the outlines unless death occurs almost immediately after the blow, before the blood has spread far into the surrounding tissue.

As a bruise gets older it changes colour, due to alteration of the haemoglobin in the extravasated blood, passing from brown, through green to yellow. Thus fresh bruises can be distinguished from bruises a week or more old, but when examining any particular bruise it is impossible to give the precise age. Bruises are common injuries and are frequently found after fights, falls and road accidents, but they are especially significant when found on the neck, suggesting throttling (see p. 130) and on the thighs of a woman, *suggesting* rape (see p. 86). They can occur as post-mortem injuries, produced by forcible blows in areas of hypostasis, e.g. the back of the scalp if the body is dropped on the ground, or on trolleys or p.m.tables.

Abrasions (grazes)

These are produced by a rough surface striking the body tangentially and removing part of the outer layer of the skin.

These injuries do not blur with the passage of time unless by healing and therefore are likely to retain a clear imprint of the surface of the object which caused them, if this has a recognisable pattern. Thus they may be of great value to the pathologist when they are found on a dead body. The tread of vehicle tyres, the patterns of belts and ropes and fingernails on the neck, and of clothing on the body may all be faithfully reproduced. A more irregular surface, such as the road, cannot leave a clear pattern but may indicate its nature by fragments of grit, etc., embedded in the raw surface of the abrasion. The direction taken by the object across the skin surface is indicated by partially detached layers of skin at the margin of the wound where the object left the skin, and by deeper linear scratches across the wound surface (Fig. 15.1).

Fig. 15.1. Direction of abrasive object over skin surface.

After death abrasions dry and their surface is liable to become dark brown and leathery, exaggerating their apparent severity, and misleading the unwary.

Lacerations (split wounds)

These are produced when a blunt object strikes the skin with sufficient force to stretch and tear it. Such wounds are commonly seen in severe crushing injuries such as occur in road accidents, and may then occur anywhere on the body. When produced by falls or blows with a weapon they are usually found in situations where the skin is easily split over bone lying close beneath it, as in the scalp or eyebrows. The object causing a lacerated wound crushes and stretches a broad area of the skin which then splits in its centre. Therefore the tissues at the margins of the split are grazed and bruised, and the edges of the wound are irregular, with strands of tougher tissue such as nerves or blood vessels stretching across the depths of the wound from one margin to the other (Fig. 15.2). When the bone is very close beneath the surface, as in the scalp, the margins of the wound may appear superficially to be clean cut, suggesting an incised wound, and close inspection will be necessary to determine its true nature.

Because of the splitting nature of the wounds they do not usually reproduce the shape of the striking object. However, fragments from its surface, such as coal dust, may be found buried in the wound.

These injuries cause true breaches of the skin, and are thus associated with bleeding, but this is less than might be expected from the size of the wound, since blood vessels are bruised and torn, and thus retract, and the blood clots readily.

Incised wounds (cuts)

These are cut or slashed wounds caused by sharp-edged agents, such as knives or razors. Since the agent is drawn across the body surface the wound is long, but shallow in relation to its length and is deeper at the end where

(a)

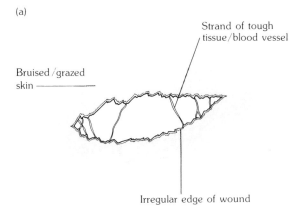

Strand of tough
tissue/blood vessel

Bruised/grazed
skin

Irregular edge of wound

(b)

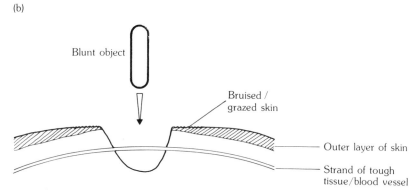

Blunt object

Bruised /
grazed skin

Outer layer of skin

Strand of tough
tissue/blood vessel

Fig. 15.2. Shape of lacerated wounds. (a) Seen from above; (b) cross-section.

the cut starts. The sharp-edged nature of the agent means that skin adjacent to the wound margin is not damaged, i.e. bruised or abraded, and the wound edges are clean cut (Fig. 15.3). The severed blood vessels bleed profusely.

The nature of the agent cannot be deduced from the wound, apart from the fact that it has a sharp cutting edge. Such wounds may be found on the neck, head and wrists in homicidal or suicidal attempts.

Stab wounds

These are penetrating injuries, whose depth within the body is much greater than the size of the wounds on the body surface. They can, of course, be produced by any long thin object which can be thrust into the body, but almost always are caused by knives. Therefore they have the same characteristics of clean-cut undamaged edges as incised wounds, and usually appear as small slits. They can be mistaken for trivial injuries because their great depth is not apparent. Moreover, they often cause little external bleeding, most of the haemorrhage occurring within the body cavities.

(a)

Undamaged margin

(b)

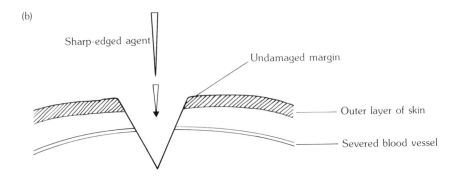

Sharp-edged agent

Undamaged margin

Outer layer of skin

Severed blood vessel

Fig. 15.3. Shape of incised wounds. (a) Seen from above; (b) cross-section.

Unlike incised injuries, stab wounds may give an indication of the shape of the weapon causing them. Thus the overall shape of the wound will generally be elliptical, but the ends of the wound may be pointed or rounded, as the edges of the blade are sharp or blunt. It may also be possible to get some idea of the dimensions of the blade from the depth of the wound and the length of the breach in the skin, but such measurements must never be regarded as precise, since an exact allowance cannot be made for the elastic recoil of the skin and subcutaneous tissues, nor for any part of the blade which may have remained outside the body. Stab wounds with unusual shapes may be caused by agents other than knives, such as screwdrivers; these can produce rectangular, or cruciform-shaped wounds.

Glass injuries

Damage caused by glass is not uncommon, especially in road accidents, and, depending on the shape and size of the fragments of glass, may consist of abrasions, incised wounds or stab wounds. The multiple abrasions and minor incised wounds caused by glass from a shattered windscreen striking the face of a person involved in a road accident are quite characteristic. Stab wounds caused accidentally by fragments of glass may have a shape which at first sight suggests that they have been caused by a knife-blade, but close examination of the margins of the wound will almost always reveal tiny side cuts due to irregularities of the glass and fragments of glass may be found embedded in the depths of the wound.

Victims of bomb explosions may bear multiple superficial injuries due to flying glass, in addition to more serious mutilations, and burns.

Interpretation of wounds

When confronted by a dead body bearing wounds the doctor will have to try to determine two things:

1   The nature of the agent or agents causing the injuries.
2   The circumstances in which the wounds occurred, i.e. accident, suicide or homicide.

Nature of agent causing injury

This can often be deduced from the nature of the wounds themselves, as suggested above, e.g. bruises, abrasions and lacerations are caused by blunt objects, such as the ground, fists, hammers, clubs, etc., incised and stab wounds by thin sharp-edged agents, e.g. knives, razor blades, spikes, etc. Abrasions may bear the pattern of the striking surface, a stab wound will reproduce to a certain extent the shape of the blade, lacerations may show the pattern of the agent and have fragments from its surface embedded in the wound margin.

Circumstances of wounding

These can often be decided, partly from the nature of the injuries, and partly from their distribution. Each individual case has to be judged on its merits, as no two cases are exactly alike, but examples of the probable findings are:

Suicidal. The injuries are usually incised or stab wounds, rarely bruises or abrasions. There are usually numerous injuries varying in severity from minor 'tentative' wounds scarcely penetrating the skin, to large and fatal injuries. It is possible for a suicidal wound, e.g. a stab or incised wound, to be solitary, but more commonly such wounds are multiple, and grouped in particular 'target' areas of the body, such as the neck, the wrists, the front of the chest on the left side. All the injuries must be in sites accessible of self-infliction.

Homicidal. Any type of injury from a bruise to a stab wound may be found, and often the body of the victim bears several types of injury. Usually the injuries are all alike in severity and 'tentative' wounds are absent. If a single homicidal wound is present, distinction from suicide or accident may be difficult, or impossible, unless such a wound occurs in a site which is inaccessible to self-infliction, e.g. a stab wound in the middle of the back could hardly be self-inflicted.

Accident. The type and distribution of injuries do not follow any particular pattern. Usually these cases are distinguished by the attendant circumstances, or the various injuries are altogether too gross to have been either

Fig. 15.4. Differences in features of cut throats. (a) Self-inflicted; (b) homicidal.

self-inflicted or due to attack by another person, e.g. a crushed head in a vehicle accident.

Examples of distinction in cut throats (Fig 15.4)

Suicidal. The wound is arranged symmetrically across the front of the neck, with irregular margins caused by repeated cuts in the same area and with tentative scratches on the skin of the neck above and below the main wound. Other groups of cuts some trivial and others deep, are likely to be found on the wrists.

Homicidal. Most often a single, deep cut, asymmetrically situated at the side of the neck. There are no tentative scratches, but deep cuts are present on the face, and also on the forearms and fingers (the latter being defence injuries caused by grasping or warding off the knife).

Accident. A single deep irregular wound with gross damage to the neck structures, fracture of the cervical spine, and with multiple fractures, lacerations and abrasions elsewhere on the body.

Internal injuries

The wounds on the surface of the body are important as indicating where and how the blows fell, and why they were sustained. But, of course, they are not usually the cause of the death, which is due to internal injuries. The following are notes on some of the commoner injuries encountered in medico-legal work.

Head injuries (Fig. 15.5)

The head is particularly the site for impacts with hard surfaces as in falls or vehicle accidents or blows with blunt objects, e.g. fists, clubs. The commonest surface injury is likely to be a laceration of the scalp.

Skull fractures

Fractures are common after such injuries, though severe and fatal intracranial injury may occur without the skull having been broken. The fractures are usually fissured, either single or in a cobweb pattern, depending on the amount of force. Depressed fractures may occur if an impact with a small area, e.g. hammer-head, occurs, and these may indicate the nature of the weapon from their shape. Fractures of the base of the skull are common, expecially from the severe forces encountered in vehicle accidents, and may be caused by force transmitted along the spine in falls on the feet or buttocks.

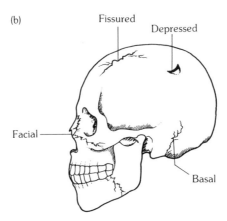

Fig. 15.5. Head injuries. (a) Intracranial haemorrhages; (b) fractures.

Intracranial haemorrhage

Extradural

Such a haemorrhage is liable to occur after a violent impact on the head, producing a fracture of the temporal region of the skull, with laceration of the middle meningeal artery as it lies in a groove in the bone. Rarely such haemorrhage may occur after a blow without a fracture of the skull, and it may be bilateral.

The particular medico-legal importance of this type of haemorrhage lies in the fact that, although treatable, there is considerable danger of its being overlooked. The impact which initiates the bleeding will usually cause temporary unconsciousness, but this is characteristically followed by a period of normal consciousness, the 'lucid interval', of one or more hours' duration, followed in turn by a recurrence of unconsciousness, due to rising intracranial pressure, and leading to death. If the patient is seen during the 'lucid interval', the doctor may not appreciate the gravity of the situation. A smell of alcohol in the patient's breath may suggest that his condition is entirely due to intoxication, with the result that he is detained in a police cell, deepening unconsciousness is mistaken for a drunken sleep, and within a few hours the patient dies.

For the safety, both of the patient and the doctor, any person who has suffered a head injury should have an X-ray examination of the skull, especially if there was a period of unconsciousness immediately after the injury, and if there is the slightest doubt about the patient's condition, even if the skull is not fractured, he should be kept under observation, and not allowed to be detained in a cell or to go home.

Subdural

These may occur from relatively slight impacts, often insufficient to cause unconsciousness and usually not producing fractures of the skull. They are particularly liable to have a slow course, first producing symptoms weeks or months after the original injury. They may occur after fights or falls, and are especially likely to be found in alcoholics and in children. In the latter, they are characteristic features of the 'battered baby', or child abuse syndrome.

Subarachnoid

These occur most commonly from the spontaneous rupture of an aneurysm of one of the basal cerebral arteries, but occasionally trauma to the head may be responsible for the rupture. It is frequently impossible to demonstrate the actual source of bleeding at autopsy. A blow on the side of the neck can rupture the vertebral artery at the base of the skull and cause a fatal subarachnoid haemorrhage from blood tracking upwards from the site of the rupture. Subarachnoid bleeding may also occur after severe brain injury, contusion or laceration. Massive haemorrhage proves rapidly fatal.

Brain damage

Blows to the head may cause bruising of the brain, both beneath the point of impact, and also at the opposite side of the head (contre-coup injury). The latter may be found at the front and sides of the head but not at the back. The actual mechanism is uncertain; there are several theories.

Greater force may cause actual laceration of the brain tissue. Haemorrhages within the brain may occur along the line of force, and may subsequently rupture on to the brain surface or into the ventricles. Such internal haemorrhages are especially dangerous when they occur in the brain stem, where they may cause rapid death from pressure on the vital centres.

Oedema of the brain may develop after head injury and may occur either localised to injured areas, or generally throughout the brain, causing prolonged unconsciousness or death.

The cause of concussion is unknown, but prolonged periods of unconsciousness after head injury, e.g. several weeks, have been found to be associated with partial demyelination.

Facial injuries

The fragile facial bones are particularly liable to damage from blows, either in vehicle accidents, or in fights, from blows with fists, or kicks. Characteristically fractures extend horizontally across the face through the orbits or across the upper jaw, and vertically downwards, from the orbits, often separating the middle third of the face from the outer two-thirds. The lower jaw may be broken in the centre, or near either angle. These injuries may prove rapidly fatal due to obstruction of the air passages by blood.

Neck injuries

Damage of the neck structures is usually found in cases of strangulation (see p. 128). Severe injuries may occur in incised wounds, or suicidal cut throats, where all the tissues may be divided down to the spine. Blows on the neck may cause rupture of the trachea with rapid onset of subcutaneous emphysema. The cervical spine may be fractured—in road accidents, due to sudden jerks of the head, at the atlanto-axial joint, or in the region of the sixth cervical vertebra.

Chest injuries

This is pre-eminently a site for stab wounds, which usually cause death by massive intrathoracic haemorrhage, the weapon having pierced the heart, the aorta, the pulmonary artery, or the venae cavae. Stab wounds of the lungs are not usually fatal, although pneumothorax occurs, unless a major pulmonary blood vessel has been severed, with consequent haemorrhage. Stab wounds of the heart are dangerous, but if the left ventricle is pierced, the thickness of the muscle wall may restrict the bleeding, allowing sufficient time for surgical treatment. A stab of the right ventricle is more rapidly fatal, blood escaping through the wound to cause haemopericardium and cardiac tamponade.

Severe impacts on the chest, as in road accidents, may fracture ribs or cause crushing injury of the lungs, with multiple small sub-pleural emphysematous blebs, or laceration of the tissue, either of the pleural surface, or confined to the interior of the lung.

In gross crushing injuries the heart may be lacerated. Uncommonly it may be bruised, but if such bruising affects a coronary artery, it may cause a traumatic coronary thrombosis within a few hours. Traumatic rupture of the aorta commonly occurs at the junction of the arch and descending parts, just beyond the origin of the left subclavian artery, and is due to violent compression of the chest. It is common in road accidents.

Fractures of the spine may be due to flexion or extension, and are usually associated with extensive injuries elsewhere.

Abdominal injuries

The abdomen is also a frequent site for stab wounds, with massive haemorrhage often resulting from perforation of the aorta or other large vessels. Alternatively transfixion of the stomach or loops of bowel may cause peritonitis.

Blows may rupture the spleen, liver or kidneys, with severe haemorrhage. More severe crushing injuries may produce gross disintegration of these organs, and rupture of hollow viscera, such as the stomach, bladder or bowel. A particular danger of such abdominal injuries is that there frequently are no signs of damage to the abdominal wall, e.g. bruising, to suggest the gravity of the condition.

Limb injuries

Lower limb injuries are frequent in accidents, notably of the upper leg in occupants of vehicles, and lower leg in pedestrians (bumper-bar fracture).

Cuts, bruises or stabs may be found on the hands or arms of victims of homicidal attacks as defence injuries from attempting to ward off blows. Their severity and irregular distribution will distinguish them from suicidal injuries, with planned sites and variation in severity.

Fractures of the neck of the femur are a common result of falls by elderly people, either due to impact with the ground, or to muscle violence when falling. These cause immobility and so predispose to death from pneumonia or venous thrombosis with pulmonary embolism.

Fractures are also associated with the hazard of fat or bone marrow embolism.

Chapter 16
Firearms

Elementary ballistics

Firearms may be considered, in the simplest form, to be of two main types:

1 Guns firing single missiles—rifles and pistols.
2 Guns firing a mass of small missiles, or shot—-shot-guns.

Rifles and pistols

These are also known as rifled weapons, after the rifling or spiral grooving of the inside of the barrel, designed to impart a spin to the missile or bullet, and so to ensure a steady flight by the gyroscopic effect produced.

Weapons with a long barrel, 2–3 feet (0.6–0.9m) long, are known as rifles. These are designed to fire the missile at a very high speed, or muzzle velocity, about 1000–4000 feet /second, and are accurate at a considerable range.

Short-barrelled weapons, 1–12 inch (25–300mm) long, are known as pistols, have a low muzzle velocity, 600–1000 feet/second, and are only accurate at relatively short range. Pistols are of two types, revolvers and automatics.

Revolvers (Fig. 16.1b) are so called because the ammunition is put in chambers in a metal cylinder which revolves before each shot to bring the next live round opposite the barrel, ready to be fired. After the bullet has been discharged the cartridge case, the brass case which contained the explosive, remains in the cylinder, and must be removed by hand.

An automatic (or self-loading) pistol (Fig. 16.1a) has the ammunition stored in a magazine, usually in the butt or handle of the gun, from which each round is fed into the barrel by a spring when the previous round has been fired. The empty cartridge case from the round that has been fired is *automatically* ejected from the pistol, landing on the ground several feet away.

The size or calibre of all these weapons is expressed as the internal diameter of the barrel, e.g. .303 inches for a rifle and .45 inches for a large pistol.

The missiles for these weapons consist of a solid metal bullet, often with a lead centre which may have a harder metal jacket. The bullet is fitted into the neck of a metal (often brass) container, the cartridge case, which contains the explosive to fire the bullet from the gun, and also a detonator, in a small copper or brass disc in the base of the cartridge case, which on

(a)

Trigger

Magazine in handle

(b)

Revolving magazine

Trigger

Fig. 16.1. (a) Automatic pistol; (b) revolver.

being struck by the hammer released by the trigger of the gun, detonates the main part of the explosive.

Most of these guns have a safety catch, a device which can lock the firing mechanism and prevent the gun being discharged accidentally.

Shot-guns

These are made for shooting game; the inside of the barrel is smooth, and the gun is designed to fire a composite missile consisting of a mass of tiny lead pellets or 'shot'.

The cartridges are loaded into the weapon by hand, and the empty cases are retained in the gun after they have been fired. The guns may have one or two barrels, side by side, or over and under, and one or two triggers, one for

Fig. 16.2. Diagrammatic cross-section of shot-gun cartridge.

each barrel. There are rarely any safety catches on hammered guns, but often on hammerless weapons.

The size or calibre may either be expressed as the inside diameter of the barrel, e.g. .410 shot-gun, or by an archaic measurement, the bore, e.g. 12-bore shot-gun. This refers to the number of balls of lead, exactly fitting the barrel, which could be made from a pound of lead.

The cartridge consists of a cardboard cylinder, with a brass base, in the centre of which is a detonator (Fig. 16.2). The cartridge contains a mass of tiny lead shot (approx. 300), each about ⅛ inch (3 mm) diameter, held in place by cardboard discs. At the bottom of the cylinder is the explosive powder, and between it and the shot is a thick cardboard disc, or wad, which functions as a piston, driving the shot before it down the gun barrel.

The shot leave the gun barrel as a solid mass, but gradually fan out during their passage through the air, so that the effect of the shot at close range is of one solid missile, at a few yards it is of a solid missile surrounded by several separate pellets, and at greater distances, it is of many separate individual pellets. The cardboard discs and the wad leave the gun with the shot, and travel for several feet before falling to the ground. Therefore in injuries caused at close range they may be found in the wound with the mass of shot.

Air-guns

These are common as adolescents' weapons, and may be of rifle or pistol type. The propellant is compressed air and the missile is a metal pellet or dart. Such weapons can be dangerous or even lethal at short ranges. Some weapons use cartridges of liquid CO_2 as the propellant, and in external appearance resemble very closely the normal revolver or automatic pistol.

Humane killers

These are specially designed for veterinary purposes for killing cattle. They may use ammunition just like normal pistols, or may be of the captive bolt type in which a metal spike is shot out of the muzzle by a blank cartridge for a few inches before being arrested.

Statutory regulations—Firearms Act 1968

Before buying a rifled weapon, i.e. a rifle or pistol, or ammunition for such a weapon, the purchaser must have a firearms certificate, obtainable from the local chief constable. The certificate relates to a particular weapon, and a variation of the certificate must be obtained for each firearm purchased.

The authority for possession of shot-guns is a shot-gun certificate, obtained in the same way as a firearm certificate, but not relating to a particular weapon.

Air-guns do not require certificates, but it is an offence to give an air-gun to a person under the age of 14, and it is illegal for a person under 17 years to have an air-gun in a public place, unless it is protected by a gun cover.

It is an offence to shorten the barrel of a shot-gun.

Firearm wounds

Bullet wounds

These are produced by a single missile travelling at high velocity. As the bullet enters the body it generally produces a round hole with clean-cut skin edges, slightly smaller than the bullet. While the missile is travelling through the body shock waves are caused, which spread laterally into the tissues, producing a large cavity in the track of the missile several times wider than the diameter of the bullet. This cavity only persists for a fraction of a second and the track of the missile within the body will be represented by a broad band of damaged tissue. The bullet will be slowed by its passage through the tissues so that if it leaves the body its exit wound will usually be an irregular split in the skin with everted edges, rather than a clean-cut hole.

The entrance wound may have special features (Fig. 16.3), dependent on the distance between the muzzle and the body when the gun is fired, for example:

1   Muzzle pressed against skin (contact injury). The gases produced by the explosion of the cartridge will enter through the skin with the missile and if they meet underlying bone, e.g. the skull, may be reflected, everting and splitting the skin at the margins of the entrance wound to produce a cruciform-shaped tear. The tissue at the margin of the wound may contain soot and powder, and carbon monoxide derived from the gases. The recoil of the gun barrel may produce a circular bruise on the skin beside the entrance wound.

2   Close range, i.e. 1–24 inches (25–600 mm). The products of explosion, i.e. the flame, soot and particles of unburnt powder, escaping from the muzzle with the missile will mark the skin around the entrance wound with a ring of blackening by soot and tattooing by fragments of unburnt powder driven into the skin. Hair may be singed.

3   Longer range, i.e. more than 2 feet (0.6 m). The gun is now too far from

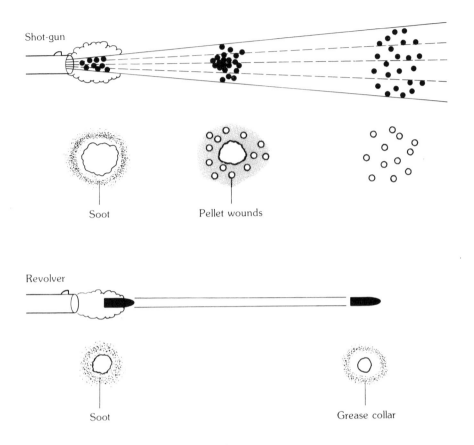

Fig. 16.3. Firearm wounds.

the skin for the products of explosion to produce any marks. Therefore, the characteristics of the entrance wound are entirely due to the bullet. As the latter penetrates the skin it inverts and abrades the margins. Therefore subsequently the wound will appear as a round hole with a band of abrasion around the margin of the hole, about $1/16$ inch (1.5 mm) broad, and outside the abrasion a rim of soiling of the skin by grease, derived from the surface of the bullet, since bullets are packed in grease as a preservative.

Thus the range of discharge of a rifled weapon can usually be determined when it is fired close to the body, but not at any range beyond about 2 feet (0.6 m).

The characteristic features of the entrance wound will usually enable it to be distinguished from the exit wound, which presents as an irregular split of the skin, with everted margins, and with no soiling of the adjacent tissues by the products of explosion. Such a distinction may be important in indicating the circumstances of the shooting; thus a contact entrance wound at the front of the head, with an exit wound at the back is consistent with suicide. A close-range entrance wound at the back of the head, with an exit wound in the forehead, on the other hand, suggests the possibility of homicide.

Shot-gun wounds

Unlike bullet wounds, it is rare for there to be an exit wound, as the shot tend to scatter within the body. The track of the missile or mass of shot within the body is broader and more ragged than is the case with a bullet.

The nature of the entrance wound (Fig. 16.3) varies with the range:

Contact injury. If the muzzle is applied to the forehead, or the roof of the mouth, the greater part of the head, including the actual entrance wound, may be destroyed.

On the trunk the wound will present as a rounded hole, with a very narrow rim of blackening by soot at the skin edges. Soot, powder and carbon monoxide will contaminate the tissues at the margins of the wound, beneath the skin.

Recoil of the gun barrel may graze or bruise the skin beside the entrance wound.

At close range—up to 1 yard (1 m). There may still be gross destruction of the head.

Elsewhere, the shot will enter the body as a solid mass, producing a round or oval hole about 1 inch (25 mm) diameter, with slightly ragged margins and with considerable blacking of the surrounding skin by soot and singeing of hair by flame unless the wound is produced through clothing. At this range the cards and wad from the cartridge will be blown into the wound along with the shot.

At intermediate ranges—about 1–4 yards (1–3.5 m). The bulk of the shot will still be travelling as a composite mass, but some individual shot pellets around the periphery will have begun to diverge. Thus the wound will appear as a central hole, with several tiny separate holes each up to ⅛ inch (3 mm) diameter, in the skin around the margin. There will be no naked eye evidence of soiling by soot or powder at this range, although traces may be found on swabs taken from the area of the wound. Cards and wad may be found in the wound.

At long range—over 4 yards (>3.5 m). As the range increases the shot will become increasingly separated and the wound at more than 10 yards (9 m) range approximately, will consist of a mass of separate tiny holes due to individual shot. Such a wound is, of course, only fatal when a shot has, for instance, punctured a main blood vessel, e.g. in the neck.

A rough indication of the range of the discharge can be obtained by measuring the diameter of the wound, from the outermost of the individual pellet wounds, in inches, and subtracting one, when the result will indicate the range in yards, e.g. wound 6 inch (1.5 cm) diameter, range 5 yards (4.5 m). This should only be used for a very rough estimate, since individual weapons vary considerably, and for greater accuracy test firings with the weapon must be made (see below).

Humane killer wounds

These may look very similar to pistol wounds, but will have a distinct circular pattern on the skin around the periphery of the hole in the entrance wound, due to the way in which the muzzle of the gun is shaped to prevent it slipping on an animal's head.

Air-gun wounds

The pellet produces a tiny hole, like the individual shot from a shot-gun. However close the range, there will be of course no soiling by soot or powder. The wounds are usually not fatal, but may be so in a child, or if the pellet injuries a large blood vessel. Although rarely fatal they are liable to produce severe injuries, e.g. the loss of an eye.

Interpretation of firearm injury

From external examination

The primary object, of course, is to distinguish between homicide, suicide and accident. For this, note must be taken of:
1   The probable type of weapon which caused the injury.
2   The site of the wound.
3   The range of discharge.
    Thus, in the case of suicide, the wound must be capable of self infliction, from its site (classically in the temple, forehead or mouth or over the heart) and the range of discharge (which must be at a range at which the deceased could reach the trigger unless some gadget has been devised to fire the gun from a distance).
    In the case of homicide, the wounds may also be in such situations, but often they are in odd sites such as the neck or the back of the body, and at longer range. They may be multiple.
    An accidental shooting may of course be by the deceased or by another, and has no features distinctive of accident. Such a case must be determined by exclusion of homicide and suicide, and by the attendant circumstances.

From autopsy

The object of the examination in addition to inspection of the surface wounds is to ascertain the direction of the missile track within the body, and the precise cause of death, and to recover the missile if this is in the body. The latter must be recovered undamaged.

A bullet may have scratches on its surface which have been produced by the barrel of the gun, and which are characteristic of that gun, so that comparison of the bullet recovered from the body with bullets fired from various weapons will enable the forensic scientist to identify the gun which was used. Similarly a cartridge case bears marks produced by the firing mechanism from which it is possible to identify the gun from which it was fired.

Therefore it is very important that all such objects, especially the missile during its removal from the body, should be treated very carefully, to avoid altering or erasing the surface markings, e.g. the ends of forceps should be wrapped in gauze before the missile is gripped.

In the case of shot-gun wounds, the cards or wads, and as much shot as possible must be collected, to determine the type of cartridge used.

If the missile cannot be easily found, then much time is saved by having the body X-rayed, since a bullet can change direction on hitting bone and end up in some very remote part of the body.

By ancillary investigations

These do not come within the province of the average doctor, but it is as well that he should know of their existence, lest he destroy the evidence vital to someone else.

Clothing. This may obviously modify the appearance of an entrance wound by trapping the soot and other products of explosion from a close-range discharge before they can reach the skin. Forensic science examination will detect them.

Discharge traces on skin. When a gun is fired some chemical traces from the discharge may be blown onto the hand holding it, and lead and nitrates may be detected by tests on swabs taken from the skin of the hand. This obviously may be useful in confirming a probable case of suicide. Therefore, the deceased's body must not be washed before these tests have been made.

Suspected weapon. Any gun found at the scene of death which could have produced the injuries will have to be examined for finger-prints and evidence of recent discharge. Furthermore the condition of the gun, e.g. well or badly maintained, and whether it is liable to accidental discharge from faulty mechanism, may be of value in determining the circumstances of the death.

Range of discharge. In cases of shot-gun injuries particularly, the range of discharge can be determined fairly accurately if the weapon is available, by firing at cardboard targets at different distances and comparing the shot patterns with the wound on the body. This allows for individual variation of weapon and ammunition, which is not possible from examination of the wound alone.

Chapter 17
Asphyxia

Definitions

Many students tend to use the words asphyxia and anoxia without being clear as to their meaning.

Anoxia means a lack of oxygen. Four different causes for this deficiency have been described:

1 Anoxic anoxia—oxygen cannot reach the blood, because there is a lack of oxygen in the lungs.

2 Anaemic anoxia—blood cannot absorb oxygen, e.g. carbon monoxide poisoning.

3 Stagnant anoxia—blood cannot carry oxygen to tissues, e.g. heart failure or embolism.

4 Histotoxic anoxia—the tissues cannot take up oxygen, e.g. cyanide poisoning.

The last three conditions are likely to be due to natural disease or to various poisons. The first, anoxic anoxia, due to lack of oxygen in the inspired air, or mechanical obstruction to respiration, is usually known as asphyxia, or mechanical asphyxia. This is the subject of this chapter and is dealt with under various headings:

Suffocation
Smothering
Choking
Crush asphyxia
Hanging
Strangulation

It must be remembered that in these various forms of mechanical asphyxia simple lack of oxygen is not the only, nor necessarily the most important factor. CO_2 accumulation may be equally disastrous, as may various cardiovascular disturbances. Together these produce the characteristic signs of asphyxia, i.e. congestion and engorgement, both externally and internally, especially of the face, with cyanosis and multiple petechial haemorrhages, most noticeable on the eyelids and skin of the face, due to rupture of capillaries from oxygen lack and raised blood pressure. The time taken for these various signs to occur depends on the circumstances, from a few seconds to several minutes.

These changes may sometimes be absent in circumstances otherwise suggestive of asphyxia, due to the occurrence of abrupt cardiac arrest (cardiac inhibition).

Cardiac inhibition

This may be a factor causing or contributing to death in any of the different kinds of mechanical asphyxia, but notably strangulation. A stimulus, such as compression, to any sensitive area, e.g. the larynx, a bronchus, or the vagus nerve itself in the neck, triggers off nerve impulses via the parasympathetic vagus nerve to the heart, which exceed the normal function of slowing the heart rate, and cause abrupt cardiac arrest. When the stimulus is associated with obstruction of the air passages, death occurs suddenly before there has been time for the normal processes of asphyxia, and their diagnostic signs, to develop.

Cardiac inhibition may occur in conditions other than mechanical asphyxia, e.g. in abortion, from blows to the abdomen, drowning, etc., in fact in any *circumstances* where violent stimulation of the parasympathetic nervous system can be caused.

Autopsy may reveal signs of the initiating cause, e.g. strangulation, but obviously cannot demonstrate the actual mechanism, which is a physiological process, by anatomical means. Diagnosis will depend on exclusion of other causes of death, and a consideration of the circumstances.

Suffocation

Death will occur if there is insufficient oxygen in the local atmosphere. Such circumstances are usually the imprisonment of the victim in a small unventilated space, e.g. in a coal mine after a roof fall, in a large safe or refrigerator, etc.

In the course of time oxygen is used up, and replaced by CO_2 and death probably occurs from the combined effects of anoxia and CO_2 narcosis and possibly heat and injuries. Under these circumstances death usually occurs only after several hours and the signs of asphyxia, i.e. cyanosis, petechial haemorrhages, etc., are especially well developed. The time actually taken to die will depend, of course, on the size of the space and the amount of available oxygen, and the needs of the victim, i.e. if he is working or is at rest.

Smothering

In this form of asphyxia the mouth and nose are obstructed. Thus a person may become smothered by heavy bedclothes, and infants may be smothered by a hand applied to the nose and mouth, by turning face down into a soft pillow, or by being overlayed by an adult's body. Putting a plastic bag over the head may cause smothering, either accidentally, in children, or deliberately as a means of suicide, in adults. Murder may be accomplished by smothering, by covering the face with a soft pillow, as in the story of the Princes in the Tower. It is a criminal offence for an adult over 16 years under the influence of alcohol to have a child under 3 in bed with him (or her), because of the danger of smothering, notably by overlaying.

The signs of asphyxia may be fully developed, but are often slight, and death is likely to be more rapid than in suffocation; choking (see below) due to inhalation of vomit caused by anoxia may accelerate the death. On occasions when the air passages are suddenly and completely obstructed as in smothering by a plastic bag, death may in fact be due to cardiac inhibition, with no signs of asphyxia.

Homicidal smothering is always difficult to diagnose, since there will probably be few, if any, marks of injury, and the signs of asphyxia are commonly only very slight. The use of an object such as a soft pillow will leave no marks or injuries to indicate the method.

Choking

Choking is caused by blockage of the air passages by foreign material. This may come from inside or outside the body.

Thus, the air passages may be blocked by inhaled vomit, by disease such as carcinoma, from falling back of the tongue during unconsciousness, or by blood or broken dentures, following facial injuries. The material may be partially masticated food, as in children or mentally defective persons or the elderly; sand, flour, etc., in industrial accidents; or cotton wool, cloth, etc., in intentional choking as a means of suicide, infanticide or homicide, or as part of a gag.

Again, signs of asphyxia may be well developed unless cardiac inhibition supervenes. The diagnosis is likely to be apparent from the history, i.e. a sudden attack of coughing and gasping with cyanosis, followed by death, and confirmed by the demonstration, at autopsy, of foreign material in the air passages. Occasionally, however, death may supervene rapidly with no signs of choking, especially when death is due to cardiac inhibition from inhaling food and such cases may be suggestive of a heart attack. They have been called 'café coronaries'.

Crush asphyxia

Crush asphyxia is due to compression of the body or chest by some heavy weight, such as a vehicle, or soil from the sides of a trench which has collapsed. The chest is compressed and the diaphragm fixed, by compression, of the abdominal wall, so that respiratory movement is impossible, and compression of the legs and abdomen forces blood into the head.

These factors produce a characteristic appearance of the victim, comprising deep engorgement and cyanosis with many large haemorrhages in the skin of the upper part of the body from the mid-chest including the shoulders and the head, and with swelling and oedema of the eyeballs, and haemorrhages into the conjunctivae.

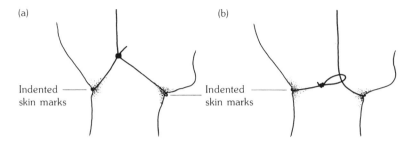

(a)   (b)

Indented — skin marks

Indented — skin marks

Fig. 17.1. Suspension by a ligature. (a) Fixed noose; (b) running noose.

Hanging

Hanging is due to compression of the neck, usually by a ligature, in such a manner that the tension is determined by the weight of the whole, or part, of the victim's body.

Hanging from a high point of suspension

In this case the victim is either fully suspended, with the feet clear of the ground, or is suspended in the standing posture, the knees slightly flexed.

Suspension is by a ligature, usually a rope, with a noose which encircles the neck. The noose may either be fixed, when the rope is knotted, or a running noose, as when the end of the rope is passed through a loop (Fig. 17.1).

The compression of the neck will produce complete closure of the blood vessels, notably the carotid arteries, and also the air passages, with resultant cerebral anoxia, unconsciousness, occurring within seconds and death within a few minutes. Signs of asphyxia are usually absent, and the face is pale and placid.

The pressure of the ligature will produce a groove or furrow in the skin of the upper part of the neck. If the ligature has a rough surface the floor of the groove will be abraded. An imprint of the surface of the ligature may be seen.

The course of the groove will depend on whether a fixed or running noose has been used. In the case of a fixed noose the side of the noose nearest to the suspending rope will be pulled upwards, assuming the shape of an inverted V. The groove in the skin will therefore have a corresponding course often with a zone of unmarked skin at the apex of the V, caused by the head falling away from the rope.

When a running noose has been used, the weight of the body will cause the noose to tighten in a mainly horizontal position. The groove will therefore also be mainly horizontal, but there may be an additional vertical mark caused by the suspending ligature.

The internal damage to neck structures is often slight compared to the depth of the skin groove. Muscles, e.g. the sternomastoids, may be ruptured, and the hyoid bone and thyroid cartilage may be broken, but bleeding at the site of these injuries is slight or absent. If the body dropped several feet before the rope tightened the cervical spine may be dislocated at the atlanto-axial joints.

The circumstances of such suspension are usually those of suicide, and this may be confirmed by the presence of suicide notes, and of a platform, such as a chair, table, etc., used to effect the suspension. The absence of such a platform and the presence of any injuries on the body apart from the mark of the ligature should be regarded with suspicion. They may indicate that the person was killed by some other means, and the body then suspended to conceal the crime.

Hanging from a low point of suspension

A comparatively slight force, about 10 lb (4.5 kg), is sufficient to occlude the blood vessels of the neck. Therefore a person can die from hanging even though the greater part of the body weight is supported by the ground, e.g. by suspension of the body in a crouching position from a door handle or bedhead.

The appearance of the body usually differs from that seen in hanging from a high point of suspension. The groove produced by the ligature is less well-marked, and may be lower on the neck and more nearly horizontal. The initial effect of the ligature is to occlude the veins, so that the face is swollen, purple in colour, with many petechial haemorrhages, i.e. the appearances are those of slow asphyxia.

Such a method may be used when full suspension is impracticable, e.g. in prison. However, it may also be used by persons curious to experience some of the effects of hanging, or may be a feature of sexual perversion, the victim being unaware that even partial occlusion of the blood vessels may cause rapid loss of consciousness. In the case of sexual perversion the deceased, always a male, may be naked or wearing female clothing and pornographic literature may be found at the scene. There may also be some soft padding, such as a handkerchief, between the ligature and the neck.

Hanging with incomplete encirclement of the neck

Hanging may occur when pressure is only applied to the front of the neck, e.g. by the arm of a chair, edge of a settee, rung of a ladder, etc. The circumstances of such hanging are almost always accidental. Marks on the neck may be indistinct or absent.

Strangulation

This is due to constriction of the neck by a force applied other than by the

(a)

Groove

(b)

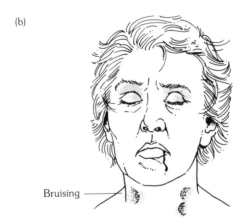

Bruising

Fig. 17.2. Differences in features of strangulation. (a) Ligature; (b) manual.

weight of the body, usually by a ligature tightened by the hands, or by the hands themselves (Fig. 17.2).

Strangulation by a ligature

The ligature. This may be any strip of pliable material, but since it will need to be something which is readily to hand, is usually either a tie or tights. The ligature may be put round the neck and the ends crossed and pulled tight, or it may be applied and knotted. The knot is usually at the front or side and may be of any kind, but the ligature should be photographed *in situ*, and then removed by cutting, without untying the knot since if it is an unusual type it may provide the police with valuable evidence. The ligature may be removed by the assailant, and strangulation must then be deduced from the marks on the neck, and distinguished from hanging.

The ligature mark. This consists of a horizontal groove around the neck, at about the level of the thyroid cartilage. It is usually much less well-marked than a hanging mark, and if a soft ligature has been used it may be almost invisible. If wire was used the mark may be deep, but very thin, and therefore difficult to see. If the ligature has been crossed and pulled tight the mark is likely to be more prominent at the site of crossover, where the two ends of the mark may be at different levels. If knotted, the ligature mark will be continuous, but broader at the site of the knot. The groove may bear the imprint of the surface of the ligature, and also on the neck there may be scratches or bruises caused by the hands of the assailant, or the hands of the victim when endeavouring to relieve the pressure.

It is necessary to avoid mistaking marks caused by tight clothing for ligature marks, and also the pallid marks found in skin folds in the fat necks of babies.

Signs of asphyxia, congestion and petechial haemorrhages are usually prominent in the head above the level of the ligature mark, but such signs may be absent where death is rapid, as by cardiac inhibition. Other injuries, such as lacerations of the scalp, stab wounds or evidence of rape, may be found in homicidal strangulation (Fig. 17.2a).

Internal injuries. Such damage usually consists of bruising of neck muscles and also fractures, particularly of the thyroid cartilage, at the level of the ligature, unless the victim is young , and the cartilage elastic. Above this level the soft tissues, especially lymph nodes and the root of the tongue, will be congested. Oedema of the lungs with foam in the air passages is frequently present.

Suicidal strangulation. This is uncommon as a method of suicide. A means of applying the ligature so that it remains in position after unconsciousness occurs is required. This may be achieved by using ligatures with rough or adhesive surfaces, by multiple loose turns round the neck, by a tourniquet mechanism, etc. Signs of asphyxia are well marked, but there is little damage to neck structures, and the ligature mark is usually only a faint band of pallor.

Accidental strangulation. In adults this is only likely to occur if clothing is caught in machinery, though it might be produced by tight clothes, e.g. collar and tie, in a person who was deeply drunk.

It is liable to happen to small children, who get entangled in pram harness or other impedimenta.

Strangulation by the hands—throttling
This form of strangulation only occurs from homicidal attempts because in

attempted self-throttling, unconsciousness would cause the hands to loosen their grip. The neck may be gripped by one or both hands, usually from the front. The external findings are bruises produced by the digits, at the front and sides of the neck, which are usually rounded and about ½ inch in diameter, but may be very faint. If the assailant has long nails these may cause scratches which present as tiny crescentic abrasions about ¼ inch long. More often the marks are indistinct, consisting only of diffuse bruising and abrasion of the skin. There are usually well-developed signs of asphyxia, and other injuries are likely to be present, e.g. bruises on the face, lacerations of the scalp, or signs of sexual interference.

The damage to the internal neck structures is likely to be more severe than in other forms of strangulation, since greater pressure can be applied in localised areas, e.g. by the thumb. Thus, extensive fractures of the hyoid bone or the thyroid and cricoid cartilages may be found, with localised, but severe bruising of the muscles (Fig. 17.2b).

The external appearances may be modified if clothing was interposed between the neck and the hands, so that in effect a partial ligature was used, and also in a rare form of strangulation, mugging, in which pressure on the neck is applied by the forearm, the assailant being behind his victim. This may leave few external signs of injury because of the broad area and soft surface of the arm.

Throttling may cause cardiac inhibition, probably due to the fact that the digits can exert localised but very deep pressure directly impinging on the vague nerve. However, this result can also occur from less severe pressure, as by a light blow or slight squeezing of the neck.

Chapter 18
Drowning

The diagnosis of drowning is a fairly common medico-legal problem. A body may be recovered from water and the doctor asked to examine it with the object of ascertaining whether or not death was due to drowning. In such a case it is unsafe to rely on the fact that the deceased has been found submerged. Death may have been due to a heart attack, during which the victim fell into the water, or the person may have been killed, e.g. by strangulation, and the body then dumped in water. If the body is badly decomposed, such diagnosis may be very difficult. Moreover, in some cases drowning may not be suspected, as when it occurs in shallow water, such as the immersion of a drunken man's face in a puddle.

The questions which the doctor may have to answer are:

1   Was death due to drowning, or to some other cause?
2   How long has the body been in the water?
3   What is the identity of the deceased?

This problem often arises in connection with drowning since the body may drift a considerable distance from the original site of entering the water and be recovered in a region where the deceased is not known. (For methods of identification, see Chapter 23.)

Cause of death in submersion

Typical drowning

During the initial struggles some water enters the air passages, and more as the body sinks. Due to the respiratory movements the water mixes with mucus and surfactant from the lungs to make a froth in the air passages. Struggling is followed by a quiescent phase, then terminal convulsions and death.

When the water is inhaled into the lungs it will affect the blood. Fresh water, i.e. from canals, rivers, etc. which is hypotonic to plasma, will enter via the pulmonary capillaries and dilute the blood, while sea-water, being hypertonic, will extract water from the blood in the pulmonary circulation, making it more concentrated (Fig. 18.1) In fresh-water drowning, water to the extent of about 2 litres may be absorbed, though in a baby 30 or 40 ml may be sufficient to cause death.

Therefore death in drowning is partly due to anoxia by exclusion of air from the lungs, but principally due to electrolyte disturbance and/or haemolysis, from the effects of the inhaled water on the blood.

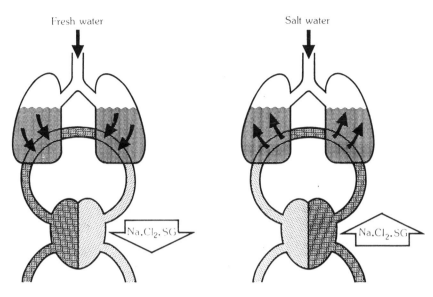

Fig. 18.1. Cause of death in drowning.

Cardiac inhibition

This is likely to occur in sudden total submersion in cold water, especially when this is unexpected, as when walking over a dock edge. Even when submersion is anticipated, e.g. at swimming-baths, a misjudged dive with sudden entry of water into the nasopharynx may cause cardiac inhibition. Death will then occur rapidly and the normal processes of drowning will not take place.

Death may also occur suddenly in people who have consumed much alcohol before entering the water.

Laryngeal spasm

This is an uncommon consequence of submersion, but entry of water into the larynx may cause severe laryngeal spasm with closure of the airway. In effect the victim dies of choking, with signs of asphyxia, which are rarely seen in typical drowning.

Appearance of the freshly drowned body

Externally the body may show signs of submersion, i.e. sodden clothing, mud-stained and wrinkled skin, etc. Hypostasis is mainly in the head and neck. The only signs indicative of drowning as opposed to submersion are the presence of fine, persistent, white foam at the nostrils and mouth, more exuding if the chest is compressed, and the presence of objects from the water, such as water weeds, tightly grasped in the hands by cadaveric spasm. Signs of asphyxia, e.g. petechial haemorrhages, etc., are not usually seen. At autopsy, the lungs will appear distended, with pallor of their surfaces, rather like asthmatic lungs, but are heavy and wet with large areas of purple mottling beneath the pleurae, and pressure from a finger will leave an indentation on the surface. The trachea and bronchi, and the cut surfaces of the lungs will contain foamy water, though occasionally all the water is absorbed, leaving the lungs dry. Water may also be present in the oesophagus and stomach, and this may contain algae or pond-weed indicating its source. Haemolysis of the blood may be apparent and may produce haemolytic staining of the wall of the aorta, not seen in the pulmonary artery. These classical signs of drowning will disappear in a few days, due to putrefaction.

Confirmatory evidence of drowning

Nature of water in the lungs

It may be necessary to distinguish water inhaled by drowning from the serous fluid in pulmonary oedema. This may be possible by microscopical examination of water in the stomach or exuding from the lung surface for algae, etc., by maceration of fragments of lung tissue in distilled water.

Biochemical tests on blood

These seek to demonstrate dilution or concentration of the blood to a different degree on each side of the heart. Thus in fresh-water drowning the blood on the left side of the heart, i.e. after passing through the lungs, will be diluted compared with that in the right side of the heart. In salt-water drowning the reverse will occur.

Such alterations can be shown by determining the specific gravities of sera from the two sides, or by determining any of the serum electrolytes, e.g. sodium or chloride ions.

These tests are only reliable if applied within about 24 hours after death, before putrefactive changes have disturbed the blood chemistry.

Diatom tests

If the water entering the blood during drowning is from such natural sources as rivers, or lakes, or the sea, it is likely to contain diatoms, and these will be distributed throughout the body by the circulation. Organs can then be removed at autopsy and all soft tissue digested with concentrated mineral acids, leaving only the acid-resistant silica shells of the diatoms. If the diatoms are discovered in such sites as the liver, brain or bone marrow this is strong evidence of drowning and is especially valuable where putrefaction has rendered useless all the other methods of making the diagnosis. However, some natural waters contain few diatoms and moreover, there is a seasonal variation in the numbers of these microscopic plants, few being present in winter.

Middle ear haemorrhages

It can be extremely helpful in establishing the diagnosis of drowning, if the middle ear on each side is removed and sections through the mastoid air cells and the middle ear itself, are made. Haemorrhages can be seen, usually by the naked eye, but on occasions it may require microscopy for confirmation. Whilst the theory is that barometric pressure is responsible, on a few occasions these haemorrhages have been seen in other forms of asphyxia, but they are almost always seen in cases of true drowning, but not when death is due to submersion as a result of a reflex cardiac arrest.

Injuries present on submerged bodies

Such injuries are relatively common, being caused after death by passing boats, by fish or aquatic mammals, or by bumping against rocks. When caused within a few hours after death, such injuries may show appreciable bruising, especially those of the head, possibly due to dilution and haemolysis of the blood, or to the distribution of hypostasis. Because of this, and the fact that wounds caused before death may be altered in appearance by the haemolysing action of the water, it may be very difficult in the case of external injuries on the body to decide whether they were caused before or after death. There should be no such difficulty, however, in regard to internal injuries, e.g. intracranial haemorrhage, damage to neck structures from throttling, etc.

Contributory factors in drowning

The autopsy in a case of drowning should be able to demonstrate any natural disease which may have caused or contributed to submersion, e.g. heart disease, cerebral infarction, etc.

Moreover, unless putrefaction has occurred, no investigation of a drowning is complete without at least a determination of the presence and the amount of any alcohol in the body.

The possibility that other drugs may be present must be remembered. This is especially important when dealing with a case of apparent drowning in a domestic bath. It has been shown that 50% of such deaths are in fact due to overdose of drugs, rather than drowning.

The possibility that the victim may have been overcome by fumes from a water heater, have suffered electrocution, or been murdered by forceable drowning or by other means and the body then put in the bath to disguise the fact, must also be considered.

Determination of period of submersion

Body temperature

Cooling is usually at approximately twice the rate in air, i.e. at about 3–4°F

(2–3°C) per hour, and the body will feel cold within a short time after submersion.

Skin changes

Whitening and wrinkling of the skin (notably of the palms and soles) occurs within a few hours. More slowly, over 1–2 weeks, the nails and hair become loosened and shed; after about 2 weeks the skin of the hands and feet is loosened, and may be stripped off. (Finger-prints may be taken from the separated skin of the fingers, or from the exposed dermis.)

Putrefaction

This, like all the other changes mentioned here, depends to a large extent on the nature and temperature of the surrounding water. Bodies in water containing hot chemical effluent from factories may show gross putrefaction in 24 hours. Otherwise the changes may be slowed down, but develop rapidly when the body is removed from the water.

Adipocere

This is likely to occur in submersion, and parts or the whole of the body may be preserved. The changes are likely to take several months to become fully developed.

Chapter 19
Physical Agents

Heat

General effects

'Heat stroke'—heat hyperpyrexia. This occurs when there is a high air temperature. The body's heat-regulating mechanism becomes overwhelmed and breaks down, especially if the usual cooling mechanism are interfered with. The body temperature rises rapidly to 107–110°F (42–44°C), the victim develops convulsions and lapses into coma and may die. In reported cases a feature at autopsy was the large number of petechial haemorrhages in the internal organs, especially the brain. This has been shown to be associated with disseminated intravascular coagulation.

This condition may occur in otherwise healthy people suddenly exposed to very high temperature, but is also a potential hazard of any drug which modifies the action of the heat-regulating mechanism, notably atropine used in premedication, especially if the patient is then exposed to a high air temperature in the theatre. A variety of malignant hyperpyrexia has recently been recognised as occurring during anaesthesia with various agents, notably halothane and suxamethonium, and due to an underlying inherited myopathy.

Heat exhaustion. This is due to prolonged exposure to hot conditions, though not as hot as those producing heat stroke. If the salt and water loss from sweating is replaced by pure water, the body becomes salt deficient, and the victim develops weakness, faintness, muscle cramps, skin rashes, etc. Replacement of the salt cures the condition, and prophylactic supplies, e.g. salt tablets, will prevent it.

Local effects—burns

The effect of local exposure of the body to heat is to produce a burn, the severity of which depends on the length of exposure and the temperature of the heat source. The minimum temperature capable of producing a burn is about 110°F (44°C) for an exposure of about 5–6 hours. Two seconds is sufficient at 150°F (65°C).

Various classifications of the severity of burns are available, the simplest being of 3 degrees:

1st degree—skin reddening and blistering.

2nd degree—whole skin destruction.

3rd degree—damage, charring etc., to tissues beneath the skin.

In addition to the depth of the burn, the other factor of importance is the surface area of the body which is affected. Twenty per cent involvement, even by superficial burns is dangerous to life.

A dead body can of course be burnt as well as a live one. Post-mortem burns can be distinguished from ante-mortem injuries by the absence of reddening of the skin at the margins, the absence of significant amounts of protein in the fluid of blisters, and the absence of microscopic evidence of inflammatory reaction.

Causes of death from burns

1 Primary (neurogenic) shock—due to pain, etc.

2 Secondary (oligaemic) shock—due to fluid loss from burned surfaces.

3 Toxaemia—absorption of various metabolites from the burnt tissue.

4 Infection, local and septicaemia.

5 Biochemical disturbances, secondary to the fluid loss, and destruction of tissue, such as hypokalaemia.

6 Acute renal failure, due to tubular necrosis.

7 Gastrointestinal disturbances—acute peptic ulcerations (Curling's ulcer), dilatation of the stomach, haemorrhage into the intestine.

8 Glottic or pulmonary oedema—due to burns of the air passages, by inhalation of flame or hot gases.

Examination of a burnt body

This usually arises when a body is found in a house or vehicle which has been the seat of a fire. The same type of considerations apply as in the case of drowning, i.e. the fact that the body is burnt and at the site of a fire is not sufficient proof that death was due to burns. The person may have died naturally, before the fire, or have been murdered, and the fire started to conceal any evidence of the crime.

Causes of death

Death in a burning building may be due to:

1 Burns.

2 Poisoning by inhaling fumes, notably carbon monoxide.

3 Injuries from falling masonry, etc.

4 Natural disease, e.g. heart failure due to coronary atheroma, precipitated by fear or exertion.

The fact that death was due to the fire may be shown by:

The burns on the surface of the body. These may show vital reaction; i.e.

reddening at the burn margin, microscopical evidence of vital reaction, etc. Moreover, the distribution of the burns on the body surface may help to show the seat of the fire, and the position of the deceased when the fire started.

The air passages. If the deceased was alive during the conflagration, the trachea, etc., will contain particles of soot adhering to the walls or embedded in viscid mucus.

The blood. In almost all cases when the deceased was alive during the fire, the blood will contain carbon monoxide derived from the fumes, often in considerable amount, e.g. up to 80% in children. The blood should always be examined for alcohol, and in appropriate circumstance for other drugs, since the findings, e.g. drunkenness, may help to explain how the fire started. Burning plastics may generate cyanide which may then be found in substantial amounts in the blood.

Special damage caused by fire

In addition to burns, damage may be produced by the action of heat on the body, living or dead, and must be distinguished from injuries caused by other means.

Pugilistic attitude. The heat causes the muscles of the limbs to stiffen and contract, so that the arms become flexed and the hands clenched, the appearance suggesting that the deceased was engaged in a fight at the moment of death.

Heat ruptures. The contraction of the skin caused by the heat may make it tear, producing large ragged wounds, resembling lacerations. When present on the scalp they can easily be mistaken for ante-mortem injuries produced by blows with a weapon. Distinction may be by their position in a burned area, and the absence of vital reaction, or bleeding.

Heat haematoma. The heat causes blood to escape from the tissues into the extradural space, where it resembles an ante-mortem injury. It may be distinguished by its position, corresponding to the site of maximum charring of the head, and the absence of other injuries, e.g. fractures of the skull.

Concealment of a crime by arson

Examination of the body may reveal bullet wounds, stab wounds, ligatures round the neck, etc., and no signs that the deceased was alive during the fire. It is unlikely that such evidence of crime will be destroyed unless damage by burning is very severe.

Scalds

The production of damage by the application of hot liquids is usually caused by accident, as when steam-pipes burst, or a child is dropped into a hot bath, or overturns a kettle. Very rarely the damage is produced deliberately, e.g. by a jealous wife, or as a means of murdering a child.

The injuries do not penetrate deeply, but may be dangerous because of the extent of body surface affected, or when affecting the upper air passages. They can be distinguished from burns by the lack of singeing of hairs.

The scald may reproduce the course taken by the hot liquid trickling over the skin, and so indicate the position of the body at the time of injury.

Cold

General effects—hypothermia

Three groups of persons are mainly at risk in this country:
1 Infants.
2 Elderly people.
3 Climbers, potholers, etc.

Infants. Cold injury may be due to inadequate clothing or heating, from poverty, or ignorance, or deliberately, and is especially liable to affect small or premature infants. For full details, textbooks of paediatrics should be consulted, but in summary the child has a good colour, and does not appear ill, but is apathetic, feels cold when touched, and possibly has patches of hardening of subcutaneous tissues.

Elderly people. These are usually living alone, with inadequate fuel or clothing, and with associated disease. e.g. myxoedema, cerebral arteriosclerosis, etc. They may be taking drugs, such as phenothiazines, or alcohol. The principal signs are pallor, mental apathy or coma, and coldness of the body. Temperatures of 90°F (32°C) or less may be recorded by special low-reading thermometers. At body temperatures below 90°F (32°C) shivering ceases, the victim does not feel cold, and the body temperature commences to fall progressively as bodily functions fail. Below 75°F (24°C) death is almost inevitable and the body temperature falls to the level of the surroundings.

At autopsy the principal signs in such persons are those of associated diseases and senility, but changes specifically due to the hypothermia may be multiple thromboses, cerebral infarction, gastric erosions, and acute pancreatitis.

Climbers, potholers, etc. Sooner or later any persons exposed to severe weather conditions may develop hypothermia, but this will be hastened by inadequate clothing, wet and windy conditions, lack of body fat, inexperience and consumption of alcohol. Fatigue is rapidly followed by exhaustion, coma, convulsions, and death. Post-mortem findings are usually non-specific, but a striking feature may be the extreme bright pink colour of the blood, resembling that seen in carbon monoxide poisoning. There may be prominent areas of purple discoloration of the limbs, especially near the joints, and multiple tiny gastric erosions.

Incapacitation by injury or drugs, especially drunkenness, may cause deaths from exposure and hypothermia, even in urban areas.

Local effects

These are described as:

1 Frostbite.
2 'Immersion foot'.

These are variations of the same condition produced by varying degrees of dry or wet cold. Slowing of the circulation is followed by damage to blood vessels, exudation and oedema, and nerve injury. Blood becomes concentrated, the circulation may cease completely and gangrene develop, especially when tissue demands for oxygen are increased by rapid reheating. In 'immersion foot' gangrene is less likely to develop, but there may be severe residual nerve and vascular damage.

Electricity

Factors in electrocution

AC current is the source of most fatalities and 50 cycles the most dangerous frequency.

Voltage. Most deaths are from supplies at about 240 volts, since that is the common domestic supply; voltages below 50 very rarely cause death. High voltages are of course dangerous, but may cause the victim to be thrown clear, while lower tensions, around 240 volts, cause muscle contraction whereby the victim holds on to the source of the current.

Amperage. This is the most important factor. Currents of 10 mA cause pain and muscle contractions, over 60 mA are dangerous, and 100 mA is fatal. Currents over 4 mA are less dangerous, e.g. high-amperage currents are used therapeutically in defibrillators.

Resistance. This may be provided by the skin, or by clothing, e.g. footwear. Dryness increases the resistance, and therefore reduces the danger. Blood has a low resistance and hence within the body, electricity tends to be conducted along blood vessels.

Earthing. Unless the victim is connected to 'earth' the current cannot flow. Therefore insulation from earth, e.g. by rubber-soled shoes, reduces the risk.

Duration of contact. Even currents of low tension may kill if the contact is prolonged.

Site of contact. Currents passing in the body across the chest, from hand to hand, or right hand to left leg, are particularly dangerous.

Causes of death
1   Ventricular fibrillation—the most important cause.
2   Respiratory failure—notably from paralysis of the muscles of respiration.
3   Central nervous system damage—usually due to contact of the source of electricity with the head.
4   Late effects—from burns or secondary haemorrhage, due to injuries caused by the current.

Post-mortem evidence

Circumstances of the death. Persons using electricity as a means of suicide will be found with wires and apparatus in position, e.g. connecting the wrists to a wall plug-socket. Accidental electrocution will usually be indicated by the position of the victims, especially when it appears that they have been making repairs to domestic appliances such as kettles, lamps, etc., or when there has been careless use of appliances, e.g. using an electric fire in a position where it can topple into a bath.

Electric mark. This is the site at which electricity enters the body and a similar mark may be found at the point of exit. Its size and distinctiveness depend on the size of the contact, the resistance of the skin, and the size of the current flowing. It usually presents as a small area of pale, hardened skin, sometimes blistered, or depressed with a raised rim, and with reddening of the adjacent skin, in fact very like a localised deep burn. If the area of contact is very large, e.g. from bath water, it is unlikely to leave any mark.

Electric burns. These are likely with very high voltages, and produce gross destruction of tissue, even charring of bone.

Internal evidence. This is likely to be sparse, and frequently non-existent.

There may be damage to the walls of blood vessels along the path of the current, or petechial haemorrhages when asphyxia has played a part in the death.

Lightning stroke

Although this also is due to the passage of electricity through the body, the appearances are different because of the very high voltage, and the blast wave produced by the discharge of electricity through the air.

Evidence at post-mortem may be:

1 Burns. These may be widespread and fan-like (called arborescent markings), due to passage of electricity over the surface of the skin, or localised to the situation of metal objects, such as wrist-watches, bracelets, buckles, etc. The metal may become magnetised. The only surface evidence may be singeing of body hairs.

2 Wounds. There may be gross wounds caused by the blast effect, with lacerations and fractures, suggesting an explosion.

3 Clothing. This may be torn or burnt or melted (e.g. nylon) or may be completely stripped from the body. At first sight this may suggest that the victim has been assaulted. Death is not inevitable from lightning stroke, but the victim may be concussed, or require artificial respiration. Sequelae may be paralyses, or mental changes, or deafness, due to rupture of the ear drum.

Radiation

Ultra-violet

The effects of this are familiar as sunburn. Severe damage may occur in unexpected circumstances where health lamps, or ultraviolet sterilisation are employed. Blindness from retinal damage is a possible hazard.

Lasers

This new form of radiation produces light rays of high energy. Its principle danger is to the eyes, where it can cause permanent blindness.

X-rays

These cause cell damage, or necrosis, and damage to blood vessels. High dosage may have local or general effects. Local burns, followed by sloughing which is very reluctant to heal, may occur. Pigmentation and scarring may follow and a late result is skin cancer.

General effects include sterility, aplastic anaemia, and deformities of the foetus *in utero*. Internal organs may develop necrosis or fibrosis, especially the kidneys (radiation nephritis).

Atomic radiation

The immediate effects of atomic explosion are intense heat and blast waves, causing burns and injuries. The effects of the damage to cells of the body produced by radiation may be 'radiation sickness', with vomiting, diarrhoea and haemorrhage occurring within a few days of exposure, or the later development of leukaemia or cachexia. The offspring of affected persons may show congenital abnormalities due to damage of the foetus *in utero*, or of the parent's germinal tissue, or sterility may develop in persons exposed to radiation.

Chapter 20
Deprivation—Starvation and Neglect

Starvation

In this country such a cause of death in adults is rare, unlike other less developed parts of the world where famine conditions occur, if crops fail. The circumstances in which a doctor is likely to see a case are:

1 As a consequence of disease preventing the taking of food, i.e. carcinoma of the oesophagus.

2 In self-neglect by the aged or mentally ill, whether from lack of money or understanding of the necessity of food.

3 As a result of accidental entombment, e.g. in a colliery accident.

4 From neglect of children or mental defectives by their parents or guardians, whether deliberately or from ignorance.

Effects of starvation

The effects of starvation depend to a certain extent on whether water is available or not. If both water and food are unavailable, death will occur in 7–10 days. If water is available, life may continue for as long as 60 days, but once 60% of the body weight has been lost, then death is almost inevitable.

The absence of food means that the body must consume its own tissues, notably protein to supply energy, and that no vitamins are available. The victim becomes emaciated, with progressive cardiac failure and with oedema and effusions into body spaces due to reduction of the plasma proteins. Frequency of urine and ketonuria occur, and there are signs of vitamin deficiency such as beriberi, pellagra, etc. Lowered resistance leads to terminal infections, broncho-pneumonia, tuberculosis, typhus, etc.

Findings at autopsy

The most striking features are emaciation of the body with almost total absence of subcutaneous or intra-abdominal fat. All the organs will be reduced in size and the walls of the intestines are very thin, while the gall-bladder is distended by bile. There may be necrosis of the liver, though probably cnly detectable microscopically, and signs of a terminal infection. There may be evidence of acute vitamin deficiency, such as scurvy or Wernicke's encephalopathy.

Neglect and cruelty

In the vast majority of cases this is a matter of neglect of children by their parents or guardians. It may take the form of:

1 Insufficient cleanliness, clothing, warmth.
2 Lack of food, or unsuitable food.
3 Mental cruelty.
4 Physical violence.

The interpretation and investigation of such a case is extremely difficult, and one of the most complicated problems in forensic medicine. The doctor has a dual role, in the early recognition and treatment among his patients, and in the examination, either of a living child, alleged to be the victim of cruelty, or of a child found dead in suspicious circumstances.

He must be extremely cautious before imputing lack of clothing, malnutrition, dirtiness, to deliberate neglect on the part of the parents. Small babies in particular may be below the normal weight for their age due to feeding problems arising from ignorance on the part of the mother, or weight loss may be due to natural disease, or the wrong type of food. Children quickly soil and damage clothes and poor families may not be able to replace them fast enough. Also children bruise easily and may sustain several surface injuries in the course of a day's play, so that the appearance of a thin, dirty, bruised, ragged child may be far more suggestive of wilful neglect than is in fact the case.

The most definitive suggestion of deliberate cruelty is likely to occur when the child is found to be suffering from a severe injury, and this is when the child will probably first be seen by the doctor. The occurrence of such cases has led to the definition of the 'Battered baby' syndrome.

Battered baby syndrome (*non-accidental injury in childhood*)

This was first described in America by a radiologist, Caffey, in 1946; the number of cases appears to have increased rapidly over the last few years.

There appear to be two types of situation in which these children present to the doctor. The child may be dead, or severely injured as a result of a single episode of violence. In this case there may be grave internal injuries, such as fractured skull with subdural haemorrhage, or a ruptured bowel or liver, associated with various fresh bruises or abrasions of the skin. The initial explanation given by the parents is that the child suffered some accident, such as a fall, but the severity of the damage is usually out of proportion to the explanation offered.

The second type of situation develops more insidiously, with minor injuries, occurring over a period of weeks or months, and leading up to the appearance of a severe injury, or death. The initial, less severe injuries, for which the child may be brought to the doctor, are often to limbs, such as a greenstick fracture of an arm. A classical site for such damage is the epiphysis of a long bone, showing on the X-ray as displacement of the epiphysis or irregularity of the epiphyseal line. A fresh epiphyseal injury may be accompanied by signs, on X-ray examination, of several other injuries of varying date, such as at other epiphyses, or of healed fractured ribs. The epiphyseal injuries in particular are caused by traction on the child's limbs, not by normal falls.

Other signs on the child's body may be multiple bruises, of different colours, suggesting different times of origin; and healing wounds, especially around the mouth where a split of the frenulum of either lip is very suggestive of a blow to the mouth. Occasionally burns may be caused by the application of lighted cigarettes or objects such as heated knives, or there may be rope marks, or linear or patterned bruises suggestive of beatings. Small rounded bruises on the head may be recognised as 'finger-tip' bruises. An unusual form of injury may be frost-bite, occurring when the child is locked up or tied in an unheated room in winter.

Internal injuries, apart from fractures, are usually deep-seated haemorrhages, around the shafts of long bones, within the skull or around the duodenum, or ruptures of viscera, especially of the liver or kidney, or of a loop of bowel, with resulting peritonitis. The typical deep injury is subdural haemorrhage. This may be due to a blow on the head, with fracture of the skull, but may occur from violent shaking of the child. It is usually associated with retinal haemorrhages. Cases have also been reported of deliberate poisoning of the child, for instance with salt.

The diagnosis of such non-accidental injury can be very difficult. Solitary injuries, or injuries occurring all at the same time may obviously have an accidental explanation. Proof of deliberate causation usually depends on demonstration of a pattern in a surface injury, indicating the agent which caused it, or on the gross disproportion between the amount of force which could be produced by the alleged accident, and the severity of the injuries found in the child.

Where there are multiple injuries of varying date, however, the problem may be easier, if they are of a type which could not be produced accidentally, and especially if any of the surface injuries, bruises or abrasions, have a pattern which enables the agent to be identified, e.g. a whip or belt, then it is almost certain that the injuries have been produced by a parent or other adult.

One should be wary of allowing apparent malnutrition or an unkempt appearance of the child to influence one's opinion on the causation of the injuries. The malnutrition may prove to be due to natural disease, and this of itself may cause the child to be more liable to fall and sustain injuries. In particular one should beware of overlooking a case of osteogenesis imperfecta, of Ehlers–Danlos syndrome, or of a haematological disorder. However, if a dead child is seen who is thin, and bruised, naturally a suspicion of cruelty will be aroused, and such cases must be referred to the Coroner.

A living child seen in hospital involves greater problems, since allegations of cruelty may be incorrect and cause the parents great suffering, yet the doctor has a duty to the child; if it is being maltreated, and is not protected, further fatal injuries may occur. It is known that once a child has been injured, there is a greater risk of it being injured again, and also of other children in the family being injured. The parents are often immature, or inadequate persons from poor social backgrounds, with a history of deprivation in their own childhood; however some battering parents are well-to-do and intelligent.

If a general practitioner suspects a patient of his is being 'battered', he would probably be wise to refer the child to hospital. This will ensure the child's immediate welfare. Apart from the paediatrician, other persons who may become involved in care of the child's welfare are the health visitor, the social worker, the NSPCC inspector, and the police. Under the Children and Young Persons Act 1969, and the Children's Act 1975, a child who is apparently being ill-treated may be taken into care or the local authority may take over parental responsibility for the child.

Cot deaths (*sudden infant death syndrome*)

This name is applied to a condition of unknown aetiology, causing about 1000 deaths each year of children between 3 and 12 months of age, though the numbers of cases are decreasing. It is of importance because the deaths are totally unexpected, and so may arouse suspicion of foul play, especially when they occur in families in poor social circumstances. The children usually are quite well on the day before death, or may have a cold. They are fed and put to bed in the evening, and are found dead in their cots in the morning, often lying face down. The subsequent autopsy examination reveals no abnormal external signs but internally there are often large petechial haemorrhages on the surface of the thymus and lungs. Histological examination shows some oedema and patchy collapse of the lungs, often with desquamation of bronchial epithelium.

The cause of the condition is unknown. A great many suggestions have been made, from overlaying and suffocation in the early days, to fulminating viral infection or allergy to milk proteins more recently. Recent suggestions have included abnormalities of cardiac conducting tissue, malfunctioning respiratory reflexes (Ondine's syndrome), hypernatraemia from incorrectly prepared feeds, abnormalities of enzymes, etc.

Recent large surveys have suggested that many of these children die of normal disease processes, demonstrable by special autopsy techniques, such as gastroenteritis but not recognised or treated in life. In another group the level of disease may appear to be barely sufficient to account for death, and it has been suggested that the significant factor is lack of parental ability to avail themselves, and their children, of available medical and social services, and perhaps lack of skill on the part of medical personnel in recognising early symptoms of disease in these children. There still remains a small group where no disease can be found. It has been suggested that these children in some way are suffering from neurological damage caused by minor birth trauma.

The existence of the 'cot death' syndrome must not cause the doctor to overlook the occasional true case of suffocation, whether accidental, from bedding or a cat, for instance, or even homicidal.

Legal protection of children

A number of laws have been framed to protect children from various hazards. The principal ones are the Children and Young Persons Act 1933 and the Children and Young Persons (Scotland) Act 1937, which define certain offences, such as:

Overlaying. It is an offence for a person over 16 years, when drunk, to take a child under 3 years of age into bed with him (or her), whereby the child dies.

Protection of fires. It is an offence if a person over 16 years, who has charge of a child under 12 years, allows the child to be in a room where the fire or heating appliance is not adequately guarded.

Neglect. Any person over 16 years, having charge of a child under that age, who assaults, ill treats, neglects, abandons, or exposes the child, in a manner likely to cause unnecessary suffering or injury, commits a misdemeanour.

Non-flammable clothing

Under the Nightdresses Safety Regulations 1967, the use of any fabric in making or trimming children's nightdresses which does not conform with specified requirements of low flammability is prohibited.

However, this does not prevent parents from buying inflammable material and making up nightdresses themselves, and the doctor, by drawing the attention of parents to the dangers of such clothing, may be able to prevent severe or fatal injury to a child.

Chapter 21
Criminal Abortion

Legal definition

The offence of criminal abortion has been defined in the Offences Against the Person Act 1861. To paraphrase, this states: A woman may commit this offence, if, being pregnant, she attempts to procure her own abortion by using any instrument, poison, or other means. Another person can be guilty if he or she attempts unlawfully to procure a woman's abortion, by any means, irrespective of whether the woman 'patient' is pregnant or not. The offence is a very grave one, carrying a maximum punishment of life imprisonment, and of course if the victim dies the abortionist will be guilty of manslaughter. In the case of a doctor who procures an abortion illegally, in addition to the punishment fixed by the statute he is almost certain to be struck off the Medical Register.

Apart from the grave offence of actively procuring an abortion, it is also an offence for a person to supply an instrument, drug, or any other thing to a woman knowing that it is to be used to procure an abortion.

In **Scotland** the offences are defined in common law and there is no comparable Act. The important point under Scottish law was that before a conviction could be achieved, it was necessary for the Crown to have proved that the woman had been pregnant.

Lawful or unlawful abortion

It is obviously important for a doctor to know whether an abortion which he feels should be performed would be considered lawful, or unlawful. Such a decision must be based on the provisions of the Abortion Act 1967. For details see Chapter 4.

Incidence of criminal abortion

Although this was once a considerable medico-legal problem, and a frequent cause of death or illness in young women, the incidence of such abortions appears to have declined markedly since the introduction of the Abortion Act. Certainly a death due to this condition is now a rarity. However the possibility remains, if the pregnant woman cannot obtain, or does not understand how to seek medical advice. Moreover there are attempts in Parliament, from time to time, to modify the law so as to make it more difficult to obtain abortions. Therefore it is still important for the doctor to be aware of the methods used, and the risks attendant upon the illegal procurement of abortion.

Methods used to procure abortion

General violence

Attempts may be made to produce abortion by taking increased and unaccustomed physical exercise, such as gardening, horse-riding, games, etc. This is very rarely effective unless an abortion was likely to occur anyway.

More dangerous is general physical violence directly applied to the body, either by the woman, e.g. throwing herself downstairs, or by another person, e.g. the father, punching and kicking the woman's body and abdomen. While unlikely to terminate the pregnancy, such violence may inflict serious injuries on the mother such as ruptured spleen.

Local violence

The object of these procedures is to dilate the cervix and dislodge the ovum so that it will be expelled. This may be achieved by:

Instruments. These range from curettes or ovum forceps, used by professional abortionists, to knitting needles and hatpins by the woman herself. In skilful hands these may be very effective and safe, but used clumsily, especially by the mother herself, they are likely to produce grave injuries of the genital tract.

Instruments, such as aspiration syringes, used in therapeutic abortion could find their way into the hands of the criminal abortionist, producing a new pattern of injuries.

Syringing. A Higginson's syringe, which may be equipped with an extra long nozzle, is used to project a jet of water containing soap or disinfectant into the vagina. The nozzle may be inserted into the cervix. The object is to drive a 'fluid wedge' between the placenta and the uterine wall, with resulting expulsion of the foetus. This is probably the most commonly used method, and is reasonably effective. Its peculiar danger is the production of an embolus of air or soap which is usually immediately fatal.

Slippery elm. An uncommon method, this consists of using a sliver of wood from the bark of a tree. This wood has the property of absorbing moisture and swelling, and when inserted into the cervix, will cause dilatation, and then induce uterine contractions, in the same way as laminaria tents which have been used in obstetrics. The main hazard is the inability to sterilise the wood, and the risk of its piercing the tissues of the genital tract.

Pastes. Various pastes can be obtained, in compressible tubes, with applicators to be inserted into the cervix. The principle, similar to the syringing method, is to force a wedge beneath the placenta. This method is effective and is used by some obstetricians. Its chief hazards are of fat embolism, or of sensitivity to the constituents of the paste, notably iodine.

Abortifacient drugs

Almost any poisonous or medicinal substance may be used by the lay person. Those commonly used are:

1 Substances supposed to increase menstrual flow. These include the typical 'old wives' remedies— purgatives such as castor oil or epsom salts; vegetable poisons like penny-royal, tansy and apiol; 'tonics', usually compound 'female' pills containing iron and quinine among other things; and corrosives, especially potassium permanganate which, used as an intra-vaginal tablet produces ulceration and so haemorrhage, resembling an inevitable abortion, which may be treated as such by an unwary doctor.

2 Substances causing uterine contraction: ergot, pituitrin, quinine and heavy metals such as lead or mercury. Quinine is particularly dangerous as it is liable to cause permanent deafness or blindness if the victim survives.

Times of using various methods

Although, of course, not rigidly applicable, there tends to be a regular sequence of the different methods employed in early pregnancy, e.g.:

1 First month—pregnancy uncertain, general violence.
2 Second month—pregnancy certain, abortifacient drugs.
3 Third month—desperation, local violence.

Dangers of abortion to the mother

General violence

Considerable violence inflicted on or by the mother may cause gross intra-abdominal or thoracic injuries, such as ruptured liver or spleen, fractured ribs or pelvis, etc., with shock and haemorrhage.

Drugs

The obvious danger is of poisoning which is likely to occur from almost any of the drugs used for this purpose, e.g. apiol may cause peripheral neuritis, penny-royal—renal tubular necrosis, quinine—cranial nerve damage, etc.

Local violence

Immediate hazards. Vagal inhibition, during dilatation of or injury to the cervix. Embolism, of air, soap or paste, during the course of syringing, or insertion of paste. Massive haemorrhage, from lacerations or penetrating wounds involving large blood vessels.

Delayed hazards (a few days). Infection, usually a fulminating clostridial septicaemia. Haemorrhage, secondary PPH. Renal tubular necrosis.

Late (1 or more weeks). Pelvic pyaemia, chronic infections, etc. Venous thrombosis, in pelvic or leg veins with danger of pulmonary embolism.

Circumstances in which a doctor may be involved in a criminal abortion

Doctor requested to perform an abortion by a patient

Directly. This may, of course, be a perfectly genuine case in which there prove to be adequate medical grounds for termination of pregnancy, under the provisions of the Abortion Act 1967. If there are no adequate medical grounds abortion must be refused but *every* effort made, by arranging financial and other assistance for the mother, to prevent her seeking unqualified assistance, and being exposed to the dangers of criminal abortion.

By guile. Thus an unknown patient may claim that she is away from home and has a retroversion in need of correction, hoping that the examination and manipulation will cause her to abort.

Doctor called to treat a patient who he discovers is suffering from the effects of a criminal abortion induced by another person

On occasions doctors have been criticised for not having informed the police in such circumstances. Therefore in 1916 the College of Physicians sought legal advice and formulated a code of conduct to be followed on such occasions:

1 The doctor must never disclose the cause of his patient's condition to anyone else without the patient's consent, unless ordered to do so in Court.

2 He should urge the patient to make a statement to the police, or, when appropriate, a dying declaration. If this is refused he should continue to treat the patient, but may seek other professional advice, medical or legal, e.g. from his medical defence society.

3 If the patient dies then the doctor must refer the case to the Coroner as being a death due to unnatural causes.

Doctor called to a sudden death due to abortion

The doctor is not likely to know that an abortion has been performed before he examines the body. An abortionist will obviously try to keep this secret. Therefore the doctor would be wise to treat all sudden deaths in women of childbearing age with suspicion until the cause has been established. When such a sudden death is due to abortion the mechanism will usually be either vagal inhibition or embolism of air or soap. Such a death will usually occur abruptly during the procedure, so that normally the body will be found where the abortion was being performed, at the patient's home or that of the abortionist.

If self-induced the general appearance of the body and its surroundings may indicate the circumstances, e.g. a body laid on the bed, legs apart, without pants, and with an instrument, or a syringe and bowl of soapy water nearby. However the victim may live long enough to clear away instruments etc., and if the abortion was performed by others they will undoubtedly have removed incriminating evidence. Then the only indication may be from the clothing, such as pants worn back to front or inside out, or a small amount of foamy fluid in the vagina, possibly smelling of disinfectant.

In such cases, as in any type of 'criminal' death, the doctor must remember to be very careful not to touch anything except the body at the scene. Vital fingerprints on instruments, bowls, glasses, etc., may otherwise be lost.

Autopsy

Although known cases of abortion will usually be the responsibility of a forensic pathologist, an unsuspected case may turn up in ordinary autopsy work.

The possibility should always be considered at any autopsy on the body of a woman of childbearing age. It is wise, in such a case, to open the abdomen first and inspect the uterus. If this is enlarged, as by pregnancy, then a careful examination must be made for signs of uterine or vaginal injury, air embolism, etc.

It is important to retain samples of right heart blood and vaginal or intra-uterine fluid for analysis for any disinfectants, etc., which may be present.

Chapter 22
Infanticide or Child Murder

At and shortly after birth a child is liable to succumb to one or other of many natural diseases. However, it is equally vulnerable to injury and whenever the dead body of a newly born infant is seen, especially if the body has been concealed, the possibility that the child had been deliberately killed must be considered. Such a killing might be murder, but under certain circumstances if done by the mother the crime will be that of infanticide or child murder.

Infanticide—the law in England and Wales

The distinction of this crime, by Act of Parliament in 1938 (the Infanticide Act), was due to an appreciation that a woman might, because of birth or lactation, be suffering from mental disturbance and so be only partly responsible for her actions—a forerunner (in England) of the doctrine of diminished responsibility.

To paraphrase the law, when a woman kills her child, provided that the child is less than 1 year old, and provided that it can be shown that at the time the woman's mental state was disturbed by the after-effects of delivery, or the effects of lactation, then the crime will not be murder, but will be infanticide. This crime is equivalent to manslaughter and is usually dealt with by putting the mother on probation.

There is no comparable statute in Scotland. There the crime is murder of a child, though similar considerations of leniency may apply in considering the mother's guilt. The killing of a newborn child is termed child murder, and as in the rest of the United Kingdom the special circumstances surrounding the death are considered with relative leniency, and usually the presence of diminished responsibility on the part of the mother is assumed to have been present at the time of the killing; the crime of child murder is thereby reduced to culpable homicide.

Circumstances involving the doctor

When any child less than 1 year old dies it may be the victim of infanticide, but the question usually arises when circumstances are suspicious, such as:

1 When a woman is found with a newly delivered dead child, especially if the child is unwanted or illegitimate, and there were no witnesses of the birth.

2 When the dead body of a newly born baby is found abandoned or concealed, with no indication of the identity of the mother.

Examination of the child

When the doctor is called upon to examine the body it is useful for him to have a scheme by which to work. This should cover three points:

1 Was the child viable?
2 Did the child have a separate existence, or was it still-born?
3 What was the cause of death, or still-birth?

Viability

This is a legal concept, not to be confused with medical terms indicating a living state, e.g. viable tissue.

It is an estimate of the unborn child's chance of survival, should it be delivered at any stage prior to full-term. The period of gestation of 28 weeks is the arbitrary point chosen. A foetus of less than 28 weeks' gestation is considered to have almost no chance of survival if born, and is called non-viable, whereas a foetus of more than 28 weeks is viable, i.e. if born it is likely to survive.

The distinction is important in law, e.g. in the crime of 'child destruction' (see below), and provides the layman with a yardstick with which to assess the evidence of a live birth in a charge of infanticide.

The maturity of a child can be assessed:

External assessment of the child's maturity

1 From the general appearance, size, and development.
2 From the weight—viable infants weigh over 2.5 lb (1 kg).
3 From the length. This is the most convenient method.

The measurement is from the crown of the head to the heel. For the first 5 months of gestation the length in cm is the square of the age, e.g. 3 months 9 cm, 4 months 16 cm. After 5 months the length in cm divided by 5, or in inches divided by 2, is the age in months, for example:

14 inches/2 = 7 months (28 weeks) = 35/5 cm.

Internal assessment of the child's maturity

At autopsy additional evidence of maturity can be obtained:

1 From the skeletal development, i.e. the occurrence of centres of ossification. These are not precise indices, but centres are likely to be present in the foot, in the talus and calcaneum at 28 weeks, at the lower end of the femur after 36 weeks, and the upper end of the tibia after 40 weeks. They can be found by direct inspection on cutting across the bone ends with a knife, or by X-ray.

2 From dental data. X-ray or dissection will show the stage of development and calcification of the teeth, and maturity can be judged from this by a dentist who is experienced in this procedure.

Separate existence

A child cannot be considered live-born unless it has shown signs of life when completely separated from the mother. This means that the whole of its body is separated, i.e. a child that is breathing when the head is delivered, but dies while one foot is still in the vagina, is in fact a still-birth. The placenta and umbilical cord do not however count as part of the body, i.e. a living child whose body is completely extruded is a live-birth, even though still attached by the umbilical cord to a placenta in the uterus.

Signs of life are defined for purposes of registration under the Births and Deaths Registration Act 1953 as breathing, beating of the heart, pulsation of the umbilical cord or definite movement of voluntary muscles.

Therefore when examining a baby's body it is necessary to show that the breathing, heart beat or movement had occurred when the child had achieved separation from the mother. It is obvious that this is always difficult, and frequently impossible, to prove. Signs to look for during examination are given in Table 22.1.

Lungs which are partially or unexpanded must be examined microscopically with the minimum of handling prior to fixation. Evidence of live-birth may then be given by the presence of hyaline membrane or pulmonary oedema, and of still-birth by findings of flooding of the lungs by amniotic fluid with squames and meconium in the alveolae, or early maceration with desquamation of bronchial epithelium. Bronchopneumonia may occur in still or live-born infants.

Note. Partial expansion of the lungs by breathing is not *proof* of separate existence; a period of breathing may occur with the child only partially delivered, if at an unattended delivery the mother collapses from pain or shock.

Putrefaction will destroy all but the most obvious signs of live-birth, i.e.

Table 22.1. Examination signs of live and still-birth.

	Live-birth	Still-birth
External examination	Separation of the umbilical cord Drying and shrivelling occurs in about 24 hours, separation in 4–5 days after birth	Maceration—this only occurs in intra-uterine death Conditions incompatible with life, e.g. gross malformation, head in a caul
Internal examination	Lungs obviously fully expanded by breathing in a recently dead baby	Gross congenital abnormalities, incompatible with life, e.g. certain forms of congenital heart disease

separation of the cord and food in the stomach. In the absence of these, the infant must be assumed to be still-born, since the contrary cannot be proved, and so the mother should be given the benefit of any doubt.

Cause of death

Once the facts of viability and separate existence have been considered, the third point—cause of death, must be decided.

Common causes of still-birth

1   Prematurity.
2   Congenital abnormalities, notably of the CVS and CNS.
3   Birth trauma—such as brain damage.
4   Anoxia—as from prolapsed cord.
5   Placental insufficiency.
6   Infection—intra-uterine pneumonia.
7   Blood disorders—erythroblastosis foetalis.

Common causes of natural neonatal death

Any of the above conditions may cause death after a period of extra-uterine existence. In addition:

1   Respiratory distress syndrome—hyaline membrane disease.
2   Cranial birth trauma—meningeal tears and intra cranial haemorrhage.
3   Infections, bronchopneumonia, umbilical sepsis with septicaemia, etc.
4   Massive pulmonary haemorrhage.

None of the conditions in these first two groups are likely to show signs by which they can be diagnosed externally.

Causes of unnatural death

Acts of omission

These are usually involuntary, due to illness or ignorance of the mother at an unattended delivery.

1   Obstruction of the airways by amniotic fluid—failure to suck out and position the child.
2   Drowning—precipitate delivery in a toilet.
3   Hypothermia—exposure after delivery, in cold weather, when no provision has been made for the birth.
4   Strangulation by the cord—failure to relieve the pressure during delivery.

Acts of commission

These are deliberate acts designed to cause the child's death:

Common

1 Suffocation. By obstruction of the nostrils and mouth by bedding, or by the mother's fingers.

2 Head injuries. By hitting the head with an object, such as a fist, or by swinging the body by the feet so as to dash the head against the wall.

Remember that fractures of the skull, cracks extending laterally from the sagittal suture, and intracranial bleeding, may occur naturally during birth. However, following deliberate injury, the injuries reflect the greater violence. There is likely to be damage, abrasion or laceration of the scalp, the fractures will be larger and probably multiple, usually with laceration of the underlying dura and laceration of the brain.

3 Strangulation. This may be by the hands, with bruising and nail scratches. Similar marks may be produced by the hands during self delivery, but are then probably distributed widely over the surface of the head, on the eyebrows, ears and the chest. Alternatively a ligature may be used, such as a piece of string. The umbilical cord may be used as the ligature and will then probably be bruised and torn by the rough handling distinguishing the circumstances from accidental strangulation by the cord during delivery. In all the circumstances the head in a recently dead baby will be congested with petechial haemorrhages on the skin and face, and there is likely to be bruising of the neck structures at autopsy.

Less common

1 Stabbing—often by some convenient agent such as (nail) scissors used to cut the cord. If a single wound it may be suggested that this occurred accidentally whilst the cord was being cut. Alternatively a sharp object such as a knitting needle may be thrust into the fontanelle, or the eye.

2 Cut throat—by scissors, a knife or a razor blade. They are often ragged with multiple wounds due to the panic of the mother.

3 Drowning—by holding the child's face in a bowl or bucket of fluid. It may be possible to prove this by finding material, such as soap, in the fluid in the lungs, otherwise it is usually impossible to distinguish from accidental drowning due to precipitate delivery. Immersion is a common mode of disposal of the body after infanticide by other means, or after still-birth.

Rare

Burning; poisoning; burial alive, etc.

All the unnatural causes of death will probably leave visible external signs, but while these may excite suspicion, it would be unwise to make a definite diagnosis without autopsy examination.

Child destruction

This crime was defined in order to bridge a gap in the law which existed between abortion and infanticide, and is set out in the Infant Life Preservation Act 1929, which applies to England and Wales only. There is no comparable statute in Scotland.

The Act makes it an offence to cause the death of a child which is unborn but viable, i.e. of 28 weeks' gestation or more while *in utero*. However, medical procedures, such as craniotomy, done to preserve the mother's life, are excluded.

Child destruction is difficult to prove, even after autopsy examination, and few are charged with this grave offence.

Concealment of birth

The law, in the Offence Against the Person Act, 1861, makes it an offence to hide a newly born child's body so as to conceal the fact of birth. It is immaterial whether the child is viable or not, whether it was live or still-born, or how it died. It is not even necessary to have discovered the child's body, if the mother can be proved to have been recently delivered. Concealment must be proved, but the criteria of this are legal, not medical matters.

It is a crime which does not carry a serious punishment, and is often charged as an alternative to infanticide. Upon conviction the woman is usually bound over, or put on probation.

In **Scotland** the Concealment of Birth (Scotland) Act 1809 applies. A woman may be convicted if she conceals her being with-child during the whole period of pregnancy and does not call for and make use of, help or assistance at the birth, and that the child be found dead or missing. Upon conviction of the crime, the woman is usually put on probation and offered psychiatric help.

Chapter 23
Identification

Identification of the living

This problem may arise in hospital when an unknown person is brought in unconscious, or when a conscious person suffers from amnesia, e.g. following a head injury. The determination of the identity of the unknown person is ultimately the responsibility of the police, but the doctor may be required to assist, by providing a detailed physical description. The main points to consider are listed below.

General appearance

For example, height, weight, sex, approximate age, colouring of skin, hair, and eyes.

Clothing

This is usually dealt with by the police, who list the clothing, examine it for laundry or other marks, and search the pockets for identifying papers, tickets, etc. Similarly all cash and jewellery must be recorded.

Finger-prints

This also is a police responsibility. The prints, of the skin ridges from the fingers, and sometimes from the palms, are taken by ink impressions on paper. The basic types of finger-print shape are arches, loops and whorls, but the patterns are so complex that no two prints from different people have ever been found to be the same, and even identical twins can be distinguished. The object of taking finger-prints from an unidentified person is so that the police can compare the prints with those on their files, of known persons, or when a possible identity has been suggested, can compare the unknown person's prints with prints on objects known to have been used by that person.

Finger-print patterns are unaltered by age, or injury, so that prints made years earlier can safely be used for comparison.

DNA profiling

A recently developed technique allows a genetic profile to be prepared from a blood, or other body tissue sample. The profile is produced by a variety of the immuno-electrophoresis technique. The resulting profile is specific to the individual, and as characteristic as are finger-prints.

Scars

These do not have the unique quality of finger-prints, for instance there must be many people alive with appendicectomy scars, but scars may be of use in distinguishing between two possible identities if only one person is known to have such a scar. Of course the greater number of scars present and the more unusual their character the more useful they will be in proving identity. Their site, exact shape and size, and approximate age must be recorded.

It should be remembered that small scars may become undetectable with age, especially linear scars from incised wounds.

Tattoos

As with scars, these are not unique, but may be very useful distinguishing features. The more elaborate and colourful the design the better, though colours fade with time, especially green and red.

Mentality

In a conscious, amnesic patient, an assessment of his ability and education maybe of value.

Anthropometry

On the Continent, systems of identification, notably the Bertillon system, have been designed which use photographs and complex measurements, especially of head shape.

The best-known medico-legal cases of identification of the living have usually involved the detection of imposters claiming estates, or the establishment of the identity of a person wrongly accused of a crime. However, such cases are rare and are very unlikely to be within the province of most doctors.

Identification of the dead

This provides one of the most fascinating aspects of forensic pathology. The problem usually arises in one of three forms:

1 A recently dead and unmutilated corpse is discovered, e.g. in a river, but with no means of identification from documents, licences, etc.

2 A body or group of bodies is gravely injured, e.g. in an aircraft crash or a fire, so that visual identification is impossible, but the size, sex, and approximate age are obvious.

3 Some grossly decomposed or skeletal human remains are discovered. The size, sex and age of the deceased cannot be determined by simple inspection of the remains.

The procedure to be adopted will obviously vary in each type of case.

Recently dead and undamaged body

When dealing with such a body it should be possible to produce a detailed description of the external appearance of the deceased, as in the case of a living person, and combine with this any evidence of natural disease, or previous injuries or operations revealed at autopsy.

Recently dead but badly damaged body

In such a case the sex, height, and approximate age of the deceased are usually readily determined by simple inspection of the body. However, the impossibility of facial recognition makes it necessary to search for other distinguishing features. These may be found in the remnants of clothing, jewellery, etc., which are present on the body, or there may be distinctive scars, tattoos or physical deformities. However, the most reliable evidence is likely to be obtained from dental investigation. An accurate dental chart should be compiled by a dentist, and may then be compared with the dental records of the various people known, for instance, to have been in the aircraft, if, as is nowadays more commonly the case, the problem of identification arises in relation to the victims of an air crash.

Most dentures nowadays have some form of identifying mark on the surface.

If a suitable blood or tissue sample can be obtained, then DNA profiling can be carried out in the same way as on the living, or blood grouping may be performed.

Skeletal remains

It is first necessary to decide whether the remains are of human origin, or the bones of some animal, and also how many individuals are represented.

If human, the problem then is to establish the primary characteristics of the deceased, i.e. sex, age, and height. Having thereby produced a bare outline of a person, the next object is to fill into this outline as many other details as possible by which the remains can be. identified.

Primary characteristics

Sex

In adults, fortunately, there are well-marked differences between the bones of the two sexes after puberty. The most useful parts of the skeleton in this respect are the pelvis (Figs. 23.1, 23.2) and the skull (Fig. 23.3).

The difference in shape of the pelvis in the two sexes can be measured by the difference of ratio between the length of pubis and the ischium, the ischio-pubic index. The index is usually less than 90 in the male, and over 90 in the female. The measurements need to be made very accurately, preferably by an anatomist.

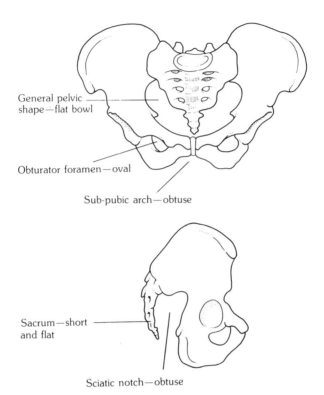

General pelvic
shape—flat bowl

Obturator foramen—oval

Sub-pubic arch—obtuse

Sacrum—short
and flat

Sciatic notch—obtuse

Fig. 23.1. Features of female pelvis.

In the case of a female, there is a well-marked groove on the front of the ilium close to its attachment to the sacrum, called the pre-auricular groove, and produced by the attachment of a ligament.

Long bones. In the male the bones are more massive, especially the articular regions, and the ridges for muscle attachment are more prominent.

Soft tissue. If the remains are only partially decomposed and not reduced to a skeleton, it may be possible from examination of soft tissue to determine the sex microscopically, by detection of the sex chromatin masses in the cell nuclei, mainly in skin or cartilage. However, this is rarely possible, due to putrefactive changes. The main value of this method is in the examination of a small part of a recently dismembered body.

Age from the bones
From soon after conception to early adult life, age is assessed from the development of ossific centres, and the fusion of these to the ends of the bones. Although the times of appearance of the ossific centres and union of epiphyses are not absolutely constant, the maximum range of variation is only of the order of 1–2 years, and therefore a reasonably reliable estimate

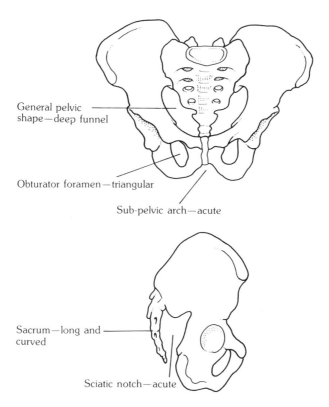

General pelvic shape—deep funnel

Obturator foramen—triangular

Sub-pelvic arch—acute

Sacrum—long and curved

Sciatic notch—acute

Fig. 23.2. Features of male pelvis.

of age can be made. It is advisable to consult textbooks or practitioners of anatomy when dealing with such a problem.

Up to 30 years the surfaces of the vertebrae bear well-marked furrows.

After 30 years age can only be approximately assessed, by the closure of skull sutures, and the onset of degenerative changes, such as osteoarthritis. Again textbooks of anatomy should be consulted for the approximate times and the variations in the closure of the skull sutures.

Age from the teeth (Fig. 23.4)

Before birth—specialised techniques exist for determining the extent of development of the teeth in the jaws, by dissection and possibly by determination of the mineral content.

In childhood—the state of eruption of the teeth of the primary or secondary dentition on direct inspection, possibly coupled with X-ray of the jaws to determine the extent of calcification of the unerupted teeth, gives a reliable indication of age, up to late adolescence.

In adults—the extent of wear of the teeth, as assessed by an experienced

(a)

(b)

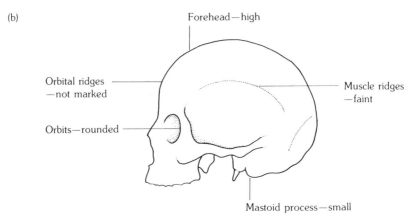

Fig. 23.3. Features of skull. (a) Male; (b) female.

(a)   (b)

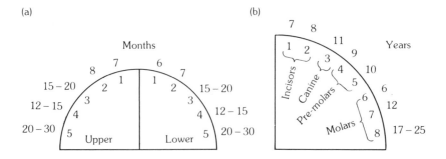

Fig. 23.4. Deduction of age from the teeth. (a) Primary dentition;
(b) secondary dentition.

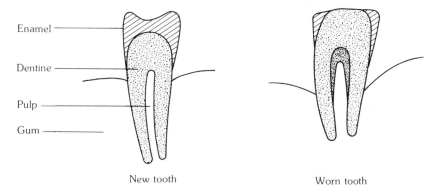

Enamel

Dentine

Pulp

Gum

New tooth   Worn tooth

Fig. 23.5. Deduction of age in adults from the wear of teeth.

dentist, on ground sections, may give some indication of age (Fig. 23.5). The method was developed first in Scandinavia by Gustafson.

Such a method can only be applied with any degree of reliability by a dentist, who has experience of its application, and even then his estimate is no more than approximate.

Height
The determination of this depends on the principle that there is a fixed relationship between the length of the limbs, especially the legs, and the total length of the body. Therefore if the length of a long bone from a limb is accurately measured and the ratio of the length of this bone, e.g. femur, to the whole body length is known, the person's height can be determined, with an accuracy of ± 1 inch (25 mm).

Tables of ratios between the length of a whole body, and the component long bones have been prepared by the examination of large numbers of cadavers, e.g. from Dupertius and Hadden's tables (for dry bones without cartilage):

Male:
Length femur × 2.238 + 69.089 cm or 27.200 in.
Length tibia × 2.392 + 81.688 cm or 32.161 in.

Female:
Length femur × 2.317 + 61.412 cm or 24.178 in.
Length tibia × 2.533 + 72.572 cm or 28.572 in.

Similar formulae are available for other bones, such as the humerus and radius, and for combinations of measurements of different bones. The measurements must be made precisely, using an osteometric board, not tape-measures, etc.

Period of interment

This can be assessed from the condition of the bones. Recent bones (e.g. 10–20 years' burial) are firm, greasy and may retain some soft tissue. Ancient bones are dry, light and brittle. Archaeological remains can be dated by the C_{14} method.

Secondary characteristics

Having determined the sex, age and height of the deceased, the next problem is to discover any additional features which may provide precise evidence of the person's identity.

Evidence of disease

Old healed fractures, operation scars on the skull, arthritis, etc. X-rays of the skeleton may be valuable. For instance, the shape of the frontal sinuses, on X-ray, is distinctive to the person. With any X-ray taken in life, there may be characteristic shapes, e.g. lipping of the spine, which can be compared with X-rays taken of the skeletal remains. In addition, in the partially decomposed body, gall-stones or uterine fibroids may be detected.

Dental evidence

Often skulls may lose teeth during putrefaction, and disinterment, or may be edentate. However, where teeth are present, an accurate record of their position, condition and any fillings, etc., should be made, preferably by a dentist. These records can then be compared with the dental records of missing persons.

Part 3
Toxicology

There is no simple classification into which all the important poisons can be fitted. This is unfortunate for the student, but the only attempt made here to classify poisons is by the circumstances of poisoning.

Chapter 24
Poisoning—General Considerations, Diagnosis and Treatment

Incidents

Poisoning as an acute cause of admission to hospital is becoming increasingly common. It is said that about 15% of admissions to hospital are from this cause. This may be due to the increasingly wide variety of medicinal products available to would be self-poisoners, and also to the increased tendency of people to indulge in self-poisoning as a means of drawing attention to domestic or psychiatric problems. It is not often appreciated that there is a considerable difference between the classes of drugs most commonly causing acute admission to hospital, and those responsible for death of patients outside hospital (Table 24.1).

Table 24.1. Differences between drugs causing admission to hospital and causing death.

Drugs commonly causing admission to hospital	Common drugs causing death as found at autopsy
Tranquillisers	Distalgesic
Salicylates	Benzodiazepines
Antidepressants	Antidepressants
Benzodiazepines	Aspirin

The frequency with which certain drugs are seen also varies with the passage of time, thus carbon monoxide was a common suicidal poison in the early 1960s, its place was later taken by barbiturates and now most recently by paracetamol.

Diagnosis

The decision that a person's illness is due to poison can be extremely difficult to make. One reason for this may be lack of suspicion in the doctor's mind, so that the possibility of poison is not even considered. Also the signs and symptoms produced by poisons are so varied, and may mimic natural disease so closely that there may be nothing in the patient's condition which is distinctive of poison. However, the sudden onset of abdominal pain with diarrhoea and vomiting or the finding of a patient who is unconscious, but with no signs of injury, should raise the possibility of poison in the doctor's mind.

Fortunately the history often indicates that poison is responsible for illness, and the nature of the poison may be known, or the tablets or liquids which have been consumed may be brought to the doctor. Otherwise, the circumstances in which poisons should be considered at the outset as a possible cause of the illness, are:

1 Sudden onset of severe illness in children.

2 Sudden illness in a person known to have been previously completely healthy, especially the sudden onset of coma.

3 Sudden illness or coma in a person suffering from depression or any mental disturbances.

4 Illness in a man whose work brings him into contact with poisonous substances, i.e. most industrial and agricultural occupations.

Even then, cases of poisoning will occur when the circumstances give no grounds for suspicion, e.g. cases of accidental domestic poisoning and unexpected suicides, especially among persons already suffering from severe disease.

Some poisons have effects which make their presence obvious, e.g. burning of the mouth by corrosives, pink coloration of the skin in carbon monoxide poisoning or grey brown due to methaemoglobin, but many poisons do not have characteristic features and present symptoms of a general nature.

Therefore, the doctor should endeavour to include the appropriate poisons in the differential diagnosis of each major symptom as suggested below. This list is not intended to be exhaustive, but to act as a guide. Students could benefit by preparing more detailed lists of their own.

Acute gastrointestinal disorder

For example, vomiting, diarrhoea and abdominal pain.

Disease	Poison
Infective gastroenteritis	Corrosives, acids,
'Acute abdomen'	alkalis, etc.
Cerebral disorders,	Irritant metals
acute infections in	and metalloids
childhood	Paraquat, paracetamol

Chronic alimentary disorders

For example, abdominal pain, constipation or diarrhoea, loss of weight and anorexia, etc.

Disease	Poison
Neoplasm	Metals, notably lead and arsenic
Ulcerative colitis	
Steatorrhoea	
Chronic infections	

Delirium

Disease	Poison
Cerebral disease, infection or haemorrhage, or tumour	Alcohols
	Antifreeze
	Volatile inhalants
Anoxic—from haemorrhage, or cardiovascular or respiratory disease	Amphetamine
	Atropine
	Cocaine, cannabis
	Lead (tetraethyl)
Pyrexia—especially in the elderly	Barbiturates
	LSD
Metabolic disorders such as uraemia, and vitamin B deficiency	Antidepressants

Coma

Disease	Poison
Cerebrovascular accidents	Barbiturates
Head injury, electric shock	Aspirin
Myxoedema, metabolic causes, e.g. diabetes, psychoses, hypothermia	Carbon monoxide
	Narcotics
	Insulin
	Alcohol
	Cyanide
	Phenol
	Tranquillisers
	Chloral
	Antidepressants

Convulsions with or without coma

Disease	Poison
Epilepsy, encephalitis	Strychnine, lead
Tetanus, hysteria	Camphor
Cerebrovascular accidents	Cocaine, atropine
	Quinine, amphetamine
	Laburnum

Acute paralysis or peripheral neuritis

Disease	Poison
Poliomyelitis	Alcohol, meths
Encephalitis	Lead, arsenic
Cerebrovascular disorders	Thallium, mercury
Diabetic neuritis	TOCP, Parathion

Motor neurone diseases	Quinine
Disseminated sclerosis	Nicotine, cyanide
Polyarteritis	Aconite
Porphyria	Hemlock

Poisoning

Alternatively, if poisoning is suspected, the likely poisons available in the particular circumstances can be considered, for example:

Common suicidal poisons
Paracetamol, antidepressants, tranquillisers, benzodiazepines.

Common household poisons
Corrosives, phenols, bleach, methyl alcohol, petrol, paraffin, creosote, polishes (containing aniline or nitrobenzene, etc.), stain removers (containing oxalate), rat poisons (dicoumarol or thallium), paraquat, dry-cleaning agents (containing carbon tetrachloride), etc.

Common industrial poisons
Gases—CO, N_2O, SO_2, $COCl_4$, H_2S, SO_2,CS_2.
Metals—lead, mercury, arsenic, antimony, chrome, beryllium, cadmium, cyanide.
Metalloids—phosphorus, and organic phosphates, fluorides.
Organic—halogenated hydrocarbons—e.g. carbon tetrachloride, trichlorethane, methyl chloride and bromide, etc.

Common poisons in childhood
Salicylates, tranquillisers, antidepressants, iron preparations, paraquat, barbiturates, lead, poisonous plants, berries, and mushrooms.

Treatment

Once poison is suspected from the clinical signs and symptoms, attempts should be made by chemical tests to determine the exact nature of the poison; this is important in case there is some specific treatment appropriate to it. However, such tests may take a considerable period of time so that urgent treatment must be instituted before the results of the tests are known and fortunately the main lines of treatment are mainly independent of the nature of the poison.

The treatment of any poisoning is basically directed by three principles:
1 Keep the patient alive—symptomatic treatment.
2 Give specific treatment, i.e. antidotes, where applicable.
3 Separate the patient from the poison.

The order in which one carries out these three lines of treatment depends on the circumstances of the individual case, and is dictated by common sense. Thus symptomatic treatment for a gaseous poison is useless while the victim remains in the contaminated atmosphere, and equally, meticulous washing out of the stomach for an ingested poison is of no avail if the patient dies of respiratory failure during the procedure.

Keeping the patient alive

This means urgent treatment to counteract the various symptoms of the poison which are threatening life.

Respiratory failure. In an unconscious patient the airway must be cleared by removal of any vomit or secretions. The insertion of an artificial airway will prevent the tongue falling backwards and obstructing the larynx. The patient must be kept in the semi-prone, 'coma' position. Initially, if breathing has ceased or is very feeble, artifical respiration, ideally by the mouth method, should be performed. In hospital adequacy of respiration should be assessed by blood-gas analysis, and if necessary a cuffed endotracheal tube passed and ventilation maintained artificially. If the arterial oxygen saturation is reduced oxygen may be given by means of a mask. In carbon monoxide poisoning hyperbaric oxygen (i.e. under increased pressure) may be used.

Circulatory failure and shock. Shock may be cured by the treatment for respiratory failure and any associated acidaemia. In addition raising the foot of the bed will increase the venous return, and may be helpful. More profound circulatory failure may be combated by the use of vasopressin agents; in addition intravenous infusions of such substances as dextran may be required but there is a danger of overloading the circulation with resulting pulmonary oedema, therefore measurements of central venous pressure must be made. Such simple measures as relief of pain, and warmth must not be forgotten.

Convulsions. Rapid sedation can be achieved by intramuscular Valium or sometimes barbiturates coupled with skilled nursing designed to reduce external stimulation to a minimum.

Coma. Skilful nursing care is the most important factor, for instance prevention of pressure sores. The patient may show hypothermia with a temperature below 95°F (35°C). Treatment may be sufficient by using insulating material to wrap the patient in, for instance metal foil blankets. With more profound cases of hypothermia active rewarming by use of a warm bath may be necessary or if more gentle measures are indicated the immersion of one limb in a bath of warm water may be adequate. Prolonged coma may result in dehydration. Measurement of electrolytes and of blood urea will be indicated, and depending on the results of these measurements appropriate fluids should be supplied by intravenous infusion.

Specific treatment

For a limited number of poisons more active measures are recommended to accelerate the elimination of the poison from the body; thus where the poison is normally excreted by the kidneys and where these are known to be functioning normally in the patient the method of forced diuresis may be appropriate. Alternatively poisons may be 'washed out' of the body by means of peritoneal dialysis or haemodialysis. Very recently methods for haemoperfusion using ion-exchange resins or animal tissues have been suggested. However all these techniques carry their own risks, for instance overloading the body with fluid, and they should only be used sparingly and with caution. In most cases they will not be needed.

Forced alkaline diuresis is of value in salicylate poisoning; intravenous infusion of 500 ml quantities of 0.9% Nacl, 5% dextrose, and 1.26% sodium bicarbonate are recommended at a rate of 2 litres of fluid per hour for about 3 hours. Forced acid diuresis is recommended for overdosage by amphetamine and quinine. In place of the bicarbonate solution ammonium chloride is used.

Peritoneal dialysis involves the passage of fluid into the peritoneal cavity through a cannula and then, after an interval, the return of the fluid. Haemodialysis involves much more complicated equipment. Both these methods are considerably affected by such factors as the amount of protein binding of the poison and so they cannot be used indiscriminately; they and the haemoperfusion techniques are only applicable to severely poisoned patients with high blood levels of the poison.

Specific antidotes are few in number and are probably the least important in the methods of treatment. Some of the effective antidotes are listed here, and details can be found under the appropriate poison.

Acid corrosives—dilute alkali (magnesia)
Alkaline corrosives—dilute acid (vinegar)
Narcotics—naloxone
Arsenic and mercury—BAL (dimercaprol)
Lead—EDTA
Copper—N-penicillamine
Iron—desferrioxamine
Cyanide—cobalt EDTA (kelo-cyanor)
Parathion—atropine and pralidoxime
Amphetamine—chlorpromazine
Paracetamol—N-acetylcysteine.

Separating the patient from the poison

The method adopted depends on the route by which the poison has been absorbed:

Inhaled gaseous poisons. Remove the patient from the contaminated atmosphere, and administer oxygen, with artificial respiration, if necessary.

Ingested poisons. If seen soon after the poison has been swallowed, provided that it is not a corrosive, or paraffin, vomiting may be produced (emesis) by putting a finger down the throat; chemical emetics that have been suggested are syrup of ipecacuanha or apomorphine hydrochloride by intramuscular injection. However each of these substances can produce its own toxic effects.

Once in hospital gastric lavage may be considered. This may be appropriate if the poison has been swallowed recently, within 4 hours, or when the poison is a salicylate or tricyclic antidepressant. It is contra-indicated where paraffin or corrosive substances have been swallowed. A stomach tube (not a Ryle's tube), should be used and small quantities—0.5–1 litre of tepid water are alternatively poured into and syphoned out of the stomach. The technique must be learnt practically in the casualty department, but one main precaution is to protect the patient's airway, by seeing that the tube is not passed into the trachea, and by positioning the patient so that the mouth is at a lower level than the lungs, and, in an unconscious patient, by passing a cuffed endotracheal tube. Recently, the use of activated charcoal, particularly given in repeated doses, has been advocated as interrupting the enterohepatic circulation.

Skin contamination. Contaminated clothing must be removed and the skin gently but adequately washed, with large amounts of warm water. No scrubbing, as this will increase absorption.

Injected poisons. If injected subcutaneously the application of ice or a tourniquet may reduce the rate of absorption. Intramuscular or intravenous injections are too rapidly absorbed to make such measures practicable.

Poisons centres

There are nowadays centres throughout the country, available to answer, by telephone, any doctor's queries regarding a case of poisoning. They should be consulted whenever any uncertainty arises, as new methods of treatment occur more rapidly than new editions of textbooks. At present they are:

Leeds Poison Information Bureau, The General Infirmary, Great George Street, Leeds LS1 3EX (Tel. 0532-430715 or 0532-432799 ext. 3547).

Poisons Information Service, New Cross Hospital, Avonley Road, London
SE14 5ER (Tel. 01-4077600 or 01-6359191).

Newcastle Poisons Information Services, Royal Victoria Infirmary, Queen
Victoria Road, Newcastle upon Tyne NE1 4LP (Tel. 091-2325131 ext.
24123 or 091-2321525 (in working hours only)).

Scottish Poisons Information Bureau, The Royal Infirmary, Edinburgh EH3
9YW (Tel. 031-2292477 or 031-2286907).

Welsh National Poisons Unit, Ward West 5, Llandough Hospital, Penarth,
Cardiff CF6 1XX (Tel. 0222-709901).

Poisons Information Centre, Royal Victoria Hospital, Grosvenor Road,
Belfast (Tel. 0232-231947 or 0232-240503 ext. 2032 (in working hours
only)).

Poisons Information Centre, Beaumont Hospital, Beaumont Road, PO Box
1297, Dublin 9 (Tel. 0001-379964 or 0001-379966).

Disposal after treatment

Many cases of attempted self-poisoning may achieve their object by the
upset caused by the attempt, but patients with more deep-seated psychiatric
problems will require referral to a psychiatrist. Children who have been
poisoned should be seen by a paediatrician.

Factors affecting action of poison

A knowledge of the relevant factors in any case of poisoning will aid the doctor in judging which methods of treatment are suitable, and in assessing the
prognosis.

Route of absorption. Thus food in the stomach may delay the action of
ingested poisons. The lethal dose of a poison by injection is usually a quarter
of the oral dose, and per rectum is twice the oral dose.

Idiosyncrasy. Rarely, in a person who is sensitive, a much smaller dose than
normal may prove fatal, e.g. in aspirin poisoning.

Age. Generally children and the aged are more susceptible to poisons, but
children can tolerate relatively more atropine than adults.

Habit. A person accustomed to taking a drug may become tolerant, and may
be able to take far more than the usual lethal dose. This appears in cases of
drug addicts, or in people on continuous therapy, e.g. epileptics.

Health. Any ill-health is likely to accelerate the effects of the poison, though
on occasion local disease, e.g. chronic gastritis may reduce its effects.

Concentration of the poison. For instance, corrosives, if diluted, may have relatively little effect, unlike pharmacologically active substances.

Chemical form. Closely similar chemical substances may differ greatly in poisonous effects, e.g. mercuric and mercurous chlorides.

Physical states. For instance a poison in liquid form will be absorbed more rapidly than the same substance in the form of a powder or tablet, from the stomach.

Dealing with a suspected case of homicidal poisoning

Poisoning is a comparatively rare method of homicide, however reported cases over the years include the use of such substances as arsenic, paraquat, insulin, morphine and barbiturates. Recently, poisoning by such substances as common salt or hypoglycaemic agents have been reported as examples of non-accidental injury in childhood.

When a doctor suspects that one of his patients is suffering from chronic poisoning, the poison being administered by another, he has a duty to protect the life of his patient, but he would be wise to refrain from voicing his suspicions until they can be confirmed.

Such confirmation can be obtained by submitting samples, e.g. blood, urine, faeces, or hair, for analysis, using some pretext to explain the procedure to the patient. However, it is simpler to send the patient to hospital, explaining one's suspicions to the physician. During the period in hospital the patient should be safe from further administration of poison, and full investigations, including analysis, can be carried out.

If the presence of poison is confirmed, the doctor would be well advised to confer with experienced colleagues, and with his medical protecton society, before informing the patient and the authorities, but obviously his guiding principle must be the welfare of his patient.

If the patient dies and poisoning is suspected to be the cause of death, then the doctor's task is relatively simple, since he must refer the case to the Coroner or the Procurator Fiscal. However, the possibility of poison should cross the doctor's mind when dealing with any sudden death. The clues may be obvious, e.g. a cup containing powder on the bedside locker, capsules in the bed, fragments of capsule or powder on the lips or in the mouth, an unusual coloration of the post-mortem staining, etc. Also the doctor should be sure that he has a record of amounts and types of drugs which he prescribed for the patient, and should see if all the drugs can be accounted for. Often the diagnosis is only made at autopsy, since it is not uncommon for there to be no external signs to suggest poisoning, and so the doctor has a duty to alert the Coroner or the Procurator Fiscal to the possibility that the sudden death of the patient may be due to poisoning, however administered.

Chapter 25
Common Suicidal Poisons

Paracetamol

As a readily available analgesic drug, this has become increasingly commonly used in suicidal attempts. Because of this, and the fact that overdosage is very dangerous as liver necrosis is likely to occur, this substance now ranks as one of the most important of suicidal poisons. Paracetamol is usually available in 500 mg tablets and severe poisoning is likely to occur if the patient has taken more than about 10 g of the drugs, i.e. 20 tablets.

The initial symptoms of poisoning soon after taking the drug are nausea, vomiting and some abdominal pain. The symptoms are not marked and may mask the gravity of the situation as severe liver failure due to hepatic necrosis is likely to occur three or four days after the drug has been consumed. This appears to be due to the fact that, whereas paracetamol is normally detoxified in the liver with glutathione, in the presence of excess amounts the available gluthathione is used up and reactive metabolites formed which then damage the liver cells, causing necrosis. Microscopical evidence of such necrosis may occur within a few hours of ingestion of the poison.

Other symptoms which may occur are damage to heart muscle causing cardiac failure, renal damage either with tubular necrosis or renal papillary necrosis, bone marrow damage with thrombocytopenia, or skin rashes. Coma may occur usually associated with liver failure.

Diagnosis

The suspicion of paracetamol ingestion may be confirmed by measurement of plasma paracetamol concentration. It has been found that liver necrosis is likely to occur if the concentration is over 300 µg/ml. It has also been shown that liver damage may be anticipated if the plasma paracetamol half-life exceeds 4 hours. This is presumably due to slowed paracetamol metabolism due to already existing liver damage.

Treatment

Current treatment aims at reducing the amount of liver damage by increasing the amount of glutathione in the liver. This is achieved by the intravenous administration of *N*-acetylcysteine. Methionine has also been used. Such treatment is only used if biochemical tests indicate the likelihood of liver damage occurring.

Other measures have been proposed, aimed at combating liver failure, such as haemoperfusion. Intravenous therapy may be required for treatment of acidosis and other biochemical abnormalities. Treatment may also be required for renal failure or massive haemorrhage, especially from the gastrointestinal tract.

Dextropropoxyphene

This substance is often one component of compound tablets mainly composed of paracetamol. It is likely to produce poisoning in its own right, with coma and convulsions and depression of respiration and cardiac function. It is also liable to lead to drug addiction. In general the symptoms resemble those of poisoning by morphine and treatment has been performed using naloxone intravenously.

Antidepressants

Typical examples of these drugs are imipramine and amitriptyline. They have anticholinergic actions preventing the destruction of catecholamines and so apparently producing cerebral stimulation. In overdosage the effects resemble those of atropine, with dry mouth, cardiac arrhythmias, hallucinations or convulsions and suppression of urine; death may result from respiratory depression. There may also be sudden and unexpected cardiac failure or cardiac arrhythmias. Serious poisoning is likely to occur if more than 1 g of the drug is taken.

Treatment

General measures to maintain life, or control convulsions, may be required. Physostigmine has been recommended as a specific treatment in the past, but because of toxic effects is not now advised by many.

Another group of drugs which was used for treatment of depression, though now much less frequently, are the mono-amine oxidase inhibitors. An example of such a drug is phenelzine (Nardil). Such drugs have been found to be dangerous if given in combination with certain other substances such as pethidine, morphine, adrenaline, and antidepressant drugs. Such combinations may result in violent hypertensive crises or sudden collapse. An acute hypertensive episode may also result if cheese, which contains tyramine, is eaten while one of these drugs is being taken.

Autopsy findings

One striking autopsy finding in cases of poisoning by tricyclic antidepressants is the very intense congestion and oedema of the lungs which feel very heavy and have a deep plum colour.

Tranquillisers

These have been classified as major tranquillisers; notably phenothiazines, and the minor tranquillisers, for instance the benzodiazepines.

An example of a phenothiazine drug is chlorpromazine (Largactil). Normal doses of a phenothiazine may produce side effects such as hyperactivity of the muscles of the head and neck, or a condition resembling Parkinson's disease. If the drug is given to a person suffering from coronary disease, postural hypotension may occur, with fatal results. Other serious side effects may be various blood disorders such as thrombocytopenic purpura or haemolytic anaemia. With some drugs liver damage and jaundice may develop, and microscopic examination reveals stasis of bile in liver cell canaliculi.

Poisoning by a large overdose may produce convulsions, succeeded by coma, with hypotension, hypothermia and cardiac arrhythmias. Treatment should be symptomatic, but avoiding analeptics and adrenaline, which may exaggerate the effect of the poison. The intravenous injection of phentolaminemesylate has been recommended for the treatment of extrapyramidal reactions.

A few cases of unexpected sudden death of patients treated with therapeutic amounts of these drugs have been reported, apparently due to abrupt heart failure. Microscopical examination has shown localised degeneration of the myocardium.

These drugs may potentiate the effects of alcohol.

Poisoning by benzodiazepines usually produces mild symptoms of drowsiness or possibly light coma which normally do not require any measures beyond general supportive treatment.

Salicylates

Source

Poisoning is usually by the readily available aspirin tablet, though it may also be caused by sodium salicylate, or soluble aspirin. Methyl salicylate liniment is also dangerous especially to children. The lethal dose is probably about 5–12 g of aspirin (i.e. 20–50 tablets) or 5–6 ml of the liniment.

Effects

Aspirin is relatively insoluble and so large amounts of powder may remain in the stomach for a long time, to be seen at autopsy. However, many analgesic tablets now available contain soluble forms of salicylate. The salicylate has an irritant effect on the stomach, causing vomiting soon after ingestion of the poison, whereby much may be returned. Within a short time the salicylate, by stimulation of the brain, causes over-breathing, acidotic in character, with sweating, dizziness and ringing in the ears. The over breathing causes disturbance of the acid–base balance of the blood, producing respiratory alkalosis, by removing CO_2. After a time there may be the development of compensatory metabolic acidosis. The electrolyte disturbances with dehydration and potassium shift are most likely to be dangerous to life. Also gastrointestinal bleeding may occur, due to the irritant action of the salicylate on mucous membranes, and from interference with the action of prothrombin. Coma is not a major feature of this variety of poisoning. Occasionally sudden death may occur before coma or dyspnoea have developed; this may be due to hypersensitivity to the drug, small amounts producing a fatal reaction. In asthmatics, aspirin may produce a fatal anaphylactic reaction.

Diagnosis

The symptoms may be misleading, as the over-breathing, with ketosis due to dehydration, may suggest diabetic or uraemic coma. On other occasions the patient may initially appear normal, in spite of being severely poisoned; sudden death may then occur unexpectedly. Ferric chloride gives a purple colour with salicylates in urine and provides a simple screening test.

Laboratory tests

Determination of the blood level of salicylate is very important as an indicator of the severity of the poisoning; when an overdose has been taken it will be over 30 mg/100 ml and levels in excess of 50 mg indicate severe poisoning. Blood electrolytes and blood pH determination is very important and serial estimations will probably need to be made, especially in children, in whom salicylate poisoning is especially dangerous.

Treatment

Gastric lavage is usually indicated, since much aspirin may remain unabsorbed in the stomach. Bicarbonate increases the excretion of salicylate in the urine, and so some should be left in the stomach, but beware of producing alkalosis. Forced alkaline diuresis has been especially recommended and is usually considered to be the treatment of choice in severe poisoning. Haemodialysis may be necessary in severe cases of poisoning, in special centres. The correction of electrolyte disturbance and dehydration is also especially important. General symptomatic treatment will be required.

Autopsy findings

The stomach will usually contain a mass of white gritty powder, with inflammation of the lining and the presence of altered blood. The only other likely findings are multiple haemorrhages on the viscera.

Barbiturates

Until recently these drugs held pride of place as being responsible for most severe cases of poisoning admitted to hospital. Now it is being found that as a cause of admission to hospital they are becoming less common and their place is tending to be taken by tricyclic antidepressants. Even as regards people dying at home before admission to hospital, paracetamol is now the commonest cause, as far as can be seen in forensic autopsy practice.

The drugs are central nervous system depressants and are used principally as hypnotics. There are many different varieties having different durations of action, for example:

1   Long action (12–24 hours)—phenobarbitone.
2   Medium action (6–8 hours)—amylobarbitone.
3   Short action (2–4 hours)—quinalbarbitone.

Ultra short-acting drugs, e.g. thiopentone, are used as anaesthetic agents. Rarely are they the cause of self-poisoning. Therapeutic doses of barbiturates are usually about 15 mg for long-acting and 150–200 mg for short-acting drugs.

Excretion is via the kidney in the case of the long-acting barbiturates; short-acting ones are detoxified in the liver.

In the case of medium and short-acting drugs about ten times the normal therapeutic dose is likely to prove fatal, i.e. 1.5–2 g.

Effects

Normal doses produce drowsiness, ataxia, and sleep. Overdoses produce an exaggeration of this, deep coma with absent reflexes, respiratory depression, peripheral circulatory failure or 'shock', loss of intestinal motility, oliguria and hypothermia.

The long-acting drugs, e.g. phenobarbitone, produce a coma which may last several days. The blood level is likely to be over 8 mg/100 ml. The danger is chiefly of infection, such as bronchopneumonia.

Short-acting drugs, e.g. seconal, produce coma lasting for about 24 hours, with blood levels above 3 mg/100 ml. The principal dangers here are of severe respiratory depression or pulmonary oedema of rapid onset. Death may occur within half an hour of consuming the drug, and may be associated with relatively low blood levels of the drug, as CO_2 retention and anoxia due to partial obstruction of the airway by the tongue will contribute to the cerebral depression.

Additive effects of other drugs

Any depressant drugs taken at the same time will add their effects to those of the barbiturates. This is particularly important in the case of alcohol, especially regarding driving. Small amounts of barbiturates, and of alcohol taken together, will have the depressant effects of marked intoxication and may produce sufficient respiratory depression to prove fatal. Thus in the presence of alcohol 0.3 to 0.6–1.0 g of amylobarbitone may prove fatal.

Laboratory tests

In a suspected poisoning, analysis of gastric washings may reveal the presence of barbiturates. Of more importance is the determination of blood levels, which may confirm the presence of barbiturate as a cause of deep unconsciousness. The actual level of barbiturate in the blood may be deceptive, as persons accustomed to taking the drug, either as a sleeping pill, or for conditions such as epilepsy, may be conscious with much higher blood levels than those normally found in cases of overdose.

Treatment

At one time active stimulation by analeptics was recommended, but nowadays it is generally considered that symptomatic treatment is the most important measure. As described on pp. 175–176, failing respiration may need to be assisted by oxygen or artificial respiration. Circulatory depression may need treatment by raising the foot of the bed. Pulmonary oedema, hypothermia, and dehydration may require appropriate treatment. Gastric lavage may be appropriate if the drug has been taken within the previous four hours. In very prolonged coma with high blood levels, haemodialysis may be necessary to reduce the amount of drug circulating and so shorten the duration of coma. There is no specific antagonist to barbiturates.

Autopsy findings

Tablets or powder residues may be found at the scene of death, for instance in cups at the bedside. There are rarely any external signs on the body, but occasionally there may be large blisters on the insides of legs and arms, or fingers, when coma has been prolonged.

Internally sodium salts of barbiturates, e.g. sodium amytal, being alkaline, may produce mild corrosion of the stomach. When taken in the form of capsules the gelatine may be found in the stomach or oesophagus, and the dye in the capsules may stain the stomach contents or linings.

Chloral

Although a reliable hypnotic, overdoses of the order of 2–10 g may be fatal with deep coma, and failure of peripheral circulation, and respiration. Gastric irritation may cause vomiting in the early stages. The drug is rapidly destroyed in the body after death, and so analysis should, if possible, be delayed for as short a time as possible. The detection chemically of even small amounts in the body may be consistent with an overdose.

Other frequently used hypnotics which may cause death from deep cerebral depression are Welldorm (dichlorphenazone), and Doriden (glutethimide).

Chapter 26
Household Poisons

Many of these substances may be found in other situations as in industry. However, poisoning by them is more likely to present as a domestic situation. Many of them are corrosive substances.

Corrosive poisons

General aspects

All corrosive poisons have in common, as their principal characteristic, chemical damage of tissues coming directly into contact with the poison. Many of them have additional systematic effects, to be considered under the various individual poisons, but their main symptoms and lines of treatment can be considered as a group.

Sites of action and effects (Fig. 26.1)

These substances are mainly colourless liquids, they either are swallowed or splash the skin. The sites likely to be affected by local contact are the skin of the face or elsewhere, the mouth and throat, the upper respiratory and alimentary tracts. The early effects are:

1 Pain and shock.
2 Vomiting.
3 Respiratory obstruction from laryngeal oedema.

Later the effects may be perforation of the stomach, or pulmonary oedema or bronchopneumonia. Late effects may be stenosis of the oesophagus, stomach or larynx or pulmonary fibrosis.

Main lines of treatment

Early

1 Pain—treat with morphine, or local anaesthetics, etc.
2 Dehydration—swallowing usually impossible, therefore i.v. fluids.
3 Corrosion—prevent further damage by neutralising poison, e.g. magnesia for acids, vinegar or very dilute acids for alkalines. Olive oil for phenol.
4 Oedema of glottis—tracheotomy.

Later

5 Oxygen, antibiotics for pulmonary oedema or infection.

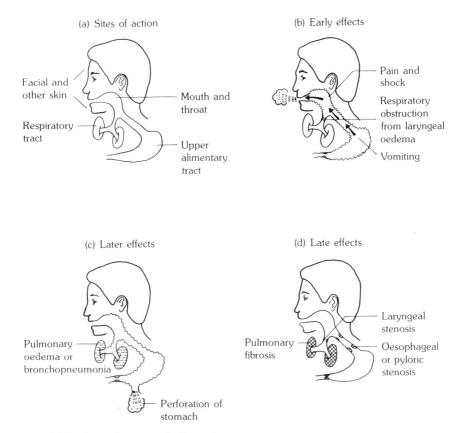

(a) Sites of action

Facial and other skin

Respiratory tract

Mouth and throat

Upper alimentary tract

(b) Early effects

Pain and shock

Respiratory obstruction from laryngeal oedema

Vomiting

(c) Later effects

Pulmonary oedema or bronchopneumonia

Perforation of stomach

(d) Late effects

Pulmonary fibrosis

Laryngeal stenosis

Oesophageal or pyloric stenosis

Fig. 26.1. Sites of action and effects of poisons.

6   Surgery for perforations and later for stenoses.

It is generally considered unwise to attempt emesis or gastric lavage in such cases of poisoning, because of the risk of perforating the alimentary tract or encouraging damage to the respiratory tract.

Individual poisons

Ammonia

Most of the few cases of corrosive poisoning which occur each year are with this substance. The circumstances may be those of suicide, but accidental poisoning occurs in industry, or when elderly persons with no sense of smell drink cleaning fluid containing ammonia.

Ammonia is a corrosive liquid with intensely irritating fumes. Therefore either the alimentary or the respiratory system may be principally affected.

If inhaled, the fumes may cause sudden cardiac inhibition and death, or after a period of coughing and choking, followed by a quiescent period, tracheo-bronchitis or pneumonia may develop. The ammonia vapour is particularly dangerous because it dissolves in the mucus of the air passages, and so its action is prolonged.

If ingested, the usual symptoms of corrosive poisoning are likely to develop. At autopsy the tissues are blackened due to the formation of alkaline haematin.

Treatment consists of neutralising with vinegar, and symptomatic measures. The initial prognosis must be cautious because of the delayed effect on the respiratory system.

Caustic alkalis

These have a more pronounced local effect than ammonia, and the damaged tissue has a slimy feel, and is grey-brown in colour at first, becoming blackened later. Since the substances, caustic soda or caustic potash do not normally occur in the form of a gas, they do not have the effects of inhalation seen in ammonia.

Neutralisation is with dilute acid, the most readily available usually being vinegar.

Acids

Usually sulphuric, hydrochloric or nitric acids. These are most likely to be a laboratory hazard, but car battery acid is strong enough to cause poisoning. Sulphuric acid in particular, extracts water, produces heat and chars and blackens the tissues. It should be neutralised with magnesia and soapy water. In the past sulphuric acid, known as oil of vitriol, was used as a weapon and thrown at enemies to cause disfigurement. It has also been used to destroy the bodies of murder victims (e.g. the notorious Haigh murder cases).

Hydrofluoric acid together with fluoride salts is principally used in industry, but may be used as a rat poison. The symptoms of poisoning are of severe gastrointestinal corrosion, and may be associated with the effects of lowered blood calcium e.g. tetany, muscle cramps, and bradycardia. Contact of the acid with the skin may cause severe devitalising burns.

Oxalic acid

This substance has important systematic as well as local effects. It is an uncommon cause of poisoning but the substance may occur at home or in industry as it is used for removing stains. Its local action, if concentrated, is corrosive to mucous membranes though not to the skin. Systemically it produces hypocalcaemia, and renal tubular damage, even in dilute solution.

The signs of poisoning will depend, therefore, on whether a large concentrated dose or a smaller dilute dose has been taken.

Large concentrated doses may cause sudden death by shock within a few minutes of ingestion. More often they produce the usual signs of corrosive poisoning, followed later by the systemic effects of hypocalcaemia and anuria.

Dilute doses will not have the corrosive effect. They may give some signs of gastrointestinal disturbance, followed in a few hours by signs of hypocalcaemia, e.g. tetany, bradycardia. Within a few days signs of renal damage, oliguria and anuria may develop.

The initial treatment is gastric lavage, with neutralisation of the oxalate by calcium salts such as calcium lactate. Symptomatic measures, possibly including haemodialysis, may be necessary.

Phenol

This substance also combines local and systemic effects. Locally grey white corrosion which is anaesthetic is produced. Phenol can be readily absorbed through the skin.

If ingested the poison causes corrosion of the alimentary tract, though with little pain, and if inhaled laryngeal and pulmonary oedema are likely to result.

Systemically, phenol acts as a fat-soluble CNS depressant, like many anaesthetic agents, and so may produce sudden collapse and coma with respiratory depression. This may occur whether absorption is through the alimentary tract, respiratory tract or skin. Treatment is symptomatic. It is important to treat skin contamination by washing and to remember the danger of inhalation of fumes from any spilt phenol. Oils, such as olive oil, may delay the absorption of phenol.

Paraquat

This substance is a herbicide, and is normally available in two products, as Gramoxone as an industrial product, or Weedol for gardeners.

It is a particulary dangerous poison in that swallowing of a small amount, even if this is unintentional and much is spat out, is liable to lead to an inevitably fatal result, after a period of several days or weeks. Estimates vary but it seems that certainly as little as 10 ml and probably substantially less may prove fatal.

Initial signs

The initial signs after swallowing the substance are those of corrosion; the victim may vomit and have abdominal pain. There is considerable soreness of the mouth and throat and the tongue may be ulcerated. If much of the substance has been swallowed the victim may then become delirious with convulsions and then comatose and respiratory failure may occur within one to three days. If a smaller amount of poison has been swallowed the victim may after a couple of days of pain, vomiting and soreness of the mouth, begin to feel much better. After a further 2 or 3 days there are likely to be signs of kidney and liver damage, with jaundice, oliguria and rising blood urea. These may then begin to improve but after about 1 week there will be the progressive onset of dyspnoea, cyanosis and respiratory distress, leading inevitably to death, within 1–3 weeks.

Confirmation of the diagnosis may be made by detection of paraquat in the urine.

Treatment

There is no specific antidote for paraquat. Attempts should be made to eliminate it from the body as rapidly and completely as possible, by emesis and lavage, and by leaving betonite or Fuller's earth in the stomach. Forced diuresis and peritoneal dialysis have been recommended and oxygen and artificial respiration may be required for the respiratory distress. Corticosteroids have been tried but without much success.

Post-mortem findings

If death occurs soon after ingestion these may consist of congestion or ulceration of the upper alimentary tract, and slight pallor of the kidneys and liver with oedema of the lungs. If survival has been for a longer period the principal signs are in the lungs which become shrunken and severely fibrotic. Microscopically the alveoli are obliterated by fibroblasts.

Ethyl alcohol

For the clinical diagnosis of drunkenness, see Chapter 11. In addition to the various alcoholic drinks, beers, wines, spirits, etc., alcohol is also available as a laboratory reagent and as a surgical or industrial spirit.

Effects

Its action in producing drunkenness by paralysis of the higher centres in the brain is described in Chapter 11. It acts as a cerebral depressant in a similar manner to an anaesthetic agent. When small amounts of alcohol are present in the body the depressant action is masked by the euphoric effect of the release of lower cerebral centres but with larger amounts depression becomes apparent, as incoordination develops, followed by coma. At very high blood levels, 400–500 mg/100 ml, medullary paralysis with failure of respiration will occur. Asphyxia from inhalation of vomit or injuries sustained during intoxication may also cause death.

Treatment

A drunken patient who is unconscious needs the same care in diagnosis and treatment as does any other victim of poisoning. He requires skilled observation and a careful differential diagnosis of the condition from other causes of coma, notably head injury. Deeply unconscious persons may need gastric lavage, maintenance of a clear airway, and possibly oxygen and assisted respiration. After a bout of very heavy drinking, followed by coma, the patient may develop hypoglycaemia and require glucose. This complication is easily overlooked.

At autopsy the body is likely to smell of alcohol. The stomach may be congested, possibly with acute erosions. The air passages may contain vomit. The possible coincidence of poisoning by other drugs must be remembered.

In the case of chronic alcoholism, the liver may show gross fatty change, or lobular cirrhosis, sometimes associated with oesophageal varices. There may be evidence of vitamin deficiencies, or malnutrition and the heart can develop an alcoholic cardiomyopathy. The ultimate cause of death is likely to be an infection.

Methyl alcohol

Source

Pure methyl alcohol is used in industry or as an antifreeze substance. In the form of methylated spirit it is mixed with ethyl alcohol, pyridine, and methyl violet. 'Meths' drinkers may be found in the vagrant community of any city, in conditions of extreme social degradation. The pyridine may give their skin a distinctive purple colour.

Effects

Methyl alcohol produces drunkenness as does ethyl alcohol, but with certain distinct differences due to the fact that metabolism of the alcohol is slow, most being excreted unchanged, and the remainder oxidised to formic acid. The effects are partly due to a direct toxic action of the methyl alcohol, but mainly to acidosis. As a result:

1 The effects are delayed, often for 24–36 hours, unless very large amounts have been taken, and early symptoms may be masked by the coincident absorption of ethyl alcohol.

2 Nausea and vomiting are associated with abdominal pain.

3 Eye signs—headache, photophobia, followed by blindness.

4 Acidosis—with rapid respiration, ketonuria, etc.

5 In heavy overdosage prolonged coma may lead to death from respiratory paralysis in 12–24 hours or more.

Treatment

Cautious administration of ethyl alcohol may prevent oxidation of methyl alcohol and so reduce the development of acidosis.

Acidosis must be treated with sodium bicarbonate, intravenously. Large amounts of fluid should be given. Morphine may be needed for pain. Gastric lavage should be performed using a solution of sodium bicarbonate. Serial estimation of blood pH will be required.

Antifreeze—ethylene glycol

Poisoning has occurred when this substance has been consumed accidentally. It has also been used as a substitute for alcohol, especially by soldiers, or in developing countries.

In the early stages cerebral symptoms are produced; later, if the patient survives, renal damage may occur. The early symptoms are drowsiness, progressing to coma, and are frequently mistaken for drunkenness. If recovery from this phase occurs, symptoms of renal damage, oliguria or anuria, may occur a few days later.

At autopsy there is evidence of nephrosis, with typical fan-shaped crystals of oxalate in the renal tubules.

Petrol and paraffin

Petrol is moderately toxic if swallowed. Inhalation of fumes produces symptoms ranging from apparent drunkenness to coma and death within minutes, depending on the concentration of the fumes. Paraffin is particular dangerous for children, who are likely to drink it. It may cause vomiting, and coma, but the principal danger is to the respiratory tract. Because of its low surface tension it can spread rapidly over the surface of bronchial mucous membranes and into the alveolar tree with widespread collapse of lung tissues. Symptoms are of dyspnoea, cough and cyanosis, followed by bronchopneumonia. X-ray films may show widely scattered opacities in the lung fields. If the child survives, severe pulmonary fibrosis may result.

As a consequence of the ability of paraffin to spread over mucous membranes it is one of the few poisons where gastric lavage is specifically contraindicated, because of the danger of soiling the upper respiratory tract. Treatment is by oxygen and antibiotics.

Chlorates and poisons causing methaemoglobinaemia

Sodium chlorate is readily available as a weed killer. Being explosive when heated with oxydisable substances, it is used in the match industry. It is rarely used as potassium chlorate in medicine as gargles and for local oral application.

Poisoning usually occurs from deliberate or accidental consumption of weedkiller. 10 g in adults may prove fatal.

Symptoms

1 Gastrointestinal upset—abdominal pain, vomiting, diarrhoea.
2 Blood—rapid and massive haemolysis, with production of Heinz bodies in red blood cells and the formation of methaemoglobin.

3 Renal damage—renal tubular obstruction following haemolysis with oliguria and anuria.

4 Hyperkalaemia—cardiovascular collapse.

Death may occur from circulatory failure, from anoxia or from uraemia. A distinctive feature, at autopsy, is likely to be chocolate-brown colour of the blood.

Methaemoglobin

Methaemoglobin has a characteristic spectrum with one band in the red region. In this substance the iron atom in the centre of the haem molecule is in the oxidised or ferric state (in normal haemoglobin the iron is in the reduced or ferrous state). Methaemoglobin does not form a loose complex with oxygen as does haemoglobin. Therefore the capacity of the blood to transport oxygen is reduced, and cyanosis and anoxia result. A characteristic 'slaty' appearance of the skin is produced, due to cyanosis and to the brown colour of the blood which is produced by methaemoglobin.

Treatment

The specific treatment of the methaemoglobinaemia consists of the reduction of ferric to ferrous iron, converting methaemoglobin to ordinary haemoglobin. The substance used is methylene blue. Usually this acts as an oxidising agent, and therefore would produce more methaemoglobin. But in low concentration in the body it is reduced by an enzyme to the colourless leuco-form, and then acts as a reducing agent, converting the iron in the blood from the ferric to the ferrous state. Treatment consists of slow intravenous administration of 25 ml of 1% solution of methylene blue.

Additional treatment includes gastric lavage, replacement of haemalysed blood by transfusion, and management of anuria.

Other substances producing methaemoglobin

Aniline in the form of marking inks, crayons, etc., may be absorbed through the skin, and has caused poisoning in babies whose nappies have been freshly marked with ink containing aniline.

Nitrobenzene is used in shoe and furniture polishes, lacquers, etc. It has been used as an adulterant of alcohol.

Nitrates may be taken in error for common salt. In country districts water derived from certain wells may contain large amounts of organic nitrates washed into the wells from chemical fertilisers on the surrounding fields. When the nitrates are ingested bacteria in the bowel convert them into nitrites, which are then absorbed and may cause poisoning. The danger is principally to recently born children in some areas; for these, supplies of pure water need to be brought in from outside the district. Poisoning has also occurred from high concentrations of nitrates in some vegetables.

Chapter 27
Industrial Poisons

Most of these substances can obviously occur in a domestic situation also. Also among them are some important homicidal poisons. Nevertheless their principal source and risk of poisoning is in industry.

Lead

Source

This metal can cause unsuspected poisoning as it can be derived from many different sources, e.g. in water which has passed through lead pipes, or in alcohol prepared or stored in vessels with a lead glaze, or from the use of battery casings for fuel, and in children who chew paint or toys which contain lead, apart from industrial processes. Poisoning is occasionally due to the accidental ingestion of soluble lead salts. Lead can also be inhaled and absorbed through broken skin (e.g. lead lotion compresses).

Effects

Acute poisoning, e.g. from drinking lead acetate solution. The symptoms are of thirst; metallic or burning taste; abdominal pains; vomiting; diarrhoea; dehydration and circulatory collapse, and possibly death (rare).

Chronic poisoning

Small amounts of lead (e.g. 0.5 mg/day) are constantly being absorbed from the environment, so that a healthy person will normally have traces of lead in his tissues, but accumulation is prevented by excretion in the urine (0.05 mg/litre) and faeces, such that a balance is maintained between ingestion and excretion.

In health the amount of lead in the blood does not exceed 0.08 mg/100 ml (0.8 μg/ml).

In chronic poisoning excessive amounts are absorbed and cannot be excreted, so that lead accumulates in the tissues, especially in the liver, kidneys and bones. The blood level rises above 0.08 mg/100 ml (0.8 μg/ml) and may reach 1.0 mg/100 ml (10 μg/ml).

The symptoms of chronic poisoning are:

General   Pallor, loss of weight
                    Anorexia and metallic taste

	Abdominal colic—relieved by pressure on abdomen
	Constipation
	Blue line on gums and anal margin
Cardiovascular	Vasoconstriction, causing pallor and hypertension
	Rarely hypertensive encephalopathy
Renal	Albuminuria, nephrotic syndrome
Locomotor	Interference with the enzymes involved in muscle contraction, therefore muscle weakness develops especially in the muscles most used, e.g. wrist-drop
Blood	Hypochromic anaemia, due to mild haemolysis and defects of haemopoesis, punctate basophilia.

Diagnosis

1 Clinically. History of exposure. Constipation, with abdominal pain, pallor, normal pulse, muscle paralysis, blue line on gums.

2 Laboratory. (a) Urine—more than 0.08 mg lead/litre of urine (24 hour samples are necessary). (b) Blood—0.08 mg lead/100 ml of blood (0.8 µg/ml). It may prove difficult from the laboratory tests to distinguish between acute and chronic lead poisoning.

The containers for the samples must be lead-free. Certain types of glass or plastic may contain traces of lead.

Treatment

Acute poisoning. Gastric lavage—with sodium or magnesium sulphate to precipitate insoluble lead sulphate and cause purgation. Parenteral treatment is by sodium calcium EDTA and dimercaprol (BAL). Abdominal colic may be relieved by pressure or calcium gluconate but morphine may be required. Convulsions can be controlled by intravenous diazepam.

Chronic poisoning. Chelating agents are used to remove the lead from the tissues, either EDTA or penicillamine.

Screening tests. For lead poisoning include detection of increased amounts of coproporphyrin and of ALA (delta-aminolaevulinic acid) in the urine. Values of coproporphyrin over 80 µg/100 mg creatinine or of ALA of 2 mg/100 mg creatinine are suggestive of lead poisoning.

Lead poisoning in children (see Chapter 29)

Lead poisoning in children is likely to present with encephalopathy and has a poor prognosis. Chronic lead poisoning is said to be responsible for some cases of mental deficiency.

Tetra-ethyl lead poisoning

This compound is used as an additive in petrol. Poisoning may occur in garage workers. Early symptoms of insomnia and mental changes may lead to delirium and mania, and death may occur from exhaustion.

Mercury

Sources

Principally an industrial poison, the metal is used in the manufacture of thermometers, explosives, etc. Mercuric chloride may be used as a disinfectant. Mercurous compounds have been used in teething powders. Organic mercury compounds are used as diuretics, and alkyl compounds as seed dressings.

Effects

Mercury may be absorbed by various routes:

1 The skin—from lotions, or the innunction of metallic mercury.

2 Ingestion—accidental swallowing of corrosive sublimate, the use of some teething powders which contain mercury, etc.

3 From the vagina, bladder, or rectum—from the use of mercury compounds as douches or antiseptic lotions.

4 Inhalation—mercury evaporates slowly at room temperature, and so the air above a pool of mercury may contain appreciable amounts of the metal. Dentists have been poisoned in this way from mercury trapped beneath the floorboards.

The action of the poison by combining with sulphydryl groups is to inhibit the action of certain enzymes. Excretion is via the kidneys, large bowel and salivary glands, and thus these organs are particularly affected by poisoning.

Acute poisoning

For example, from swallowing corrosive sublimate. Severe irritant symptoms occur, abdominal pain, diarrhoea and vomiting together with salivation, and 1 or 2 days later nephrosis and anuria may develop.

Chronic poisoning

Usually occurs from industrial exposure.

Symptoms

1 *Ptyalism*—persistent salivation and infection of the mouth and gums with loosening of the teeth.

2 *Tremor*—coarse and jerky, of small muscles such as those of the hands.

The condition was once known as 'Hatter's Shakes', from the use of mercury in the fur felting industry.

3 *Erethism*—emotional disturbances, e.g. irritability, with insomnia and excessive timidity or anger.

4 *Renal damage*—nephrosis and uraemia.

5 General effects—such as emaciation, gastrointestinal disorders, etc.

Special forms of poisoning

Alkyl mercury poisoning. From eating treated seeds or from the vapour. The main effects are on the nervous system, with ataxia and dysarthria and restriction of visual fields. Large outbreaks have occurred in some underdeveloped countries. Disease has also occurred from accumulation of mercury in foodstuffs, such as fish, derived from contamination by effluent from industrial plant (Minimata Bay disease).

Pink disease. Rarely seen now. It occurred from poisoning of children by mercury compounds in teething powders. The children were miserable, with muscle weakness and skin rashes, and reddening of the hands and feet.

Mercurial diuretics. Intravenous injection has caused sudden collapse and death, though not specifically due to the mercury content.

Treatment

Acute poisoning requires gastric lavage. Egg albumin will precipitate the poison and must then be removed by lavage. Symptomatic treatment will be necessary, such as for anuria. The specific antidote for acute or chronic mercury poisoning is BAL. Penicillamine has also been found of value.

Thallium

As yet a rare poison in this country; its use as a depilatory in the treatment of ringworm was discontinued in 1930. Abroad it is a constituent of rat pastes, and has been used as a homicidal poison, for which its properties are almost ideal.

It produces abdominal pain and vomiting, after a delay of 12–24 hours. The illness continues over the next 2–3 weeks with peripheral neuritis, cerebral symptoms, disturbances of sleep, and a rash, and death may occur from respiratory or cardiac failure. A most striking sign is the sudden and almost total loss of body hair.

Barium

Barium sulphate, as used in X-ray examinations, is harmless, but barium carbonate or chloride are toxic, and so poisoning may occur from the mistaken use of the wrong substance, or from accidental contamination of food, e.g. by flour containing barium sulphate, prepared as a rat poison.

The symptoms are of gastrointestinal irritation, i.e. pain and vomiting, and of stimulation followed by paralysis of muscle fibres with muscle twitching and convulsions followed by respiratory and cardiac arrest.

Chromium

Chronic poisoning in industry produces ulcers in the skin and nasal septum (chrome holes). Ingestion of chromates causes severe gastrointestinal irritation, followed by kidney damage and anuria.

Cadmium

The danger is chiefly from the inhalation of the fumes. These have a necrotising action on alveolar membranes, with severe pulmonary oedema, followed, if the victim survives, by pulmonary fibrosis.

Beryllium

This substance produces chronic granulomas, if inhaled or introduced into the skin through cuts. Severe pulmonary fibrosis can result.

Zinc

Inhalation of fumes can cause inflammation of the lungs and bronchopneumonia. Ingestion of zinc sulphate or chloride will cause intense gastrointestinal irritation, and possibly corrosion.

Cyanide

Sources

Solid sodium and potassium cyanides are used in industrial processes, and are readily available for use in various hobbies, e.g. photography. Hydrogen cyanide gas is used for fumigation. Liquid hydrogen cyanide (prussic acid) is used in industry and by veterinary surgeons and is an ingredient of certain medicines.

Effects

Cyanide inhibits the oxidising enzyme, cytochrome oxidase, and prevents the uptake of oxygen by the cells.

As a result the blood remains fully oxygenated, so that both arterial and venous blood have a uniform bright red colour. The lethal amount of prussic acid is about 2 ml, and of alkaline cyanide about 300 mg.

The consumption of such a quantity of cyanide is often followed by collapse and death within seconds, but on occasions death may be delayed for many minutes, the victim being in deep coma with almost undetectable pulse and respiration, and in such cases the specific treatment may save the victim's life.

Treatment

This is one of the few poisons where specific antidote is really important in treatment, and when available should precede all other measures. The antidotes consist of amyl nitrite, dicobalt edetate (kelocyanor) and sodium thiosulphate. The amyl nitrite in the form of a capsule should be broken into a handkerchief and inhaled by the victim. If he has ceased to breath then artificial respiration, but *not* by mouth to mouth method should be performed.

Kelocyanor should be injected as 300 mg in 20 ml of glucose solution intravenously and slowly over 3–4 minutes. Such injection may cause anaphylactic reaction and cardiac arrythmia if given too fast. Kelocyanor may produce prompt revival of the victim; if not then 50 ml of 50% sodium thiosulphate solution should be given by slow intravenous injection. The injections can be repeated if recovery is not apparent within 10 minutes. A mixture of solutions of ferrous sulphate and sodium carbonate may act as an antidote to swallowed cyanide in the stomach. Kelocyanor is toxic if cyanide has not been taken.

Autopsy findings

The bitter-almond smell of cyanide may be apparent at the scene of death or when examining the body, but many people are unable to detect the odour. The hypostasis may be bright red, due to the oxygenated blood, but the appearance can be confused with carbon monoxide poisoning or exposure of the body to cold.

Internally, the organs will also be bright red in colour. Sodium or potassium cyanide may degenerate with time to produce ammonia and sodium or potassium hydroxide, therefore poisoning with these substances may produce the signs of corrosive poisoning in the alimentary tract, and may cause the stomach to smell of ammonia.

Organo-phosphorus compounds

Source

These are used in agriculture as insecticides in the form of sprays or dusts. The compound which is best known as a poison is parathion, which is common as a suicidal or homicidal poison on the Continent, but in this country the only cases reported have been accidental. There are many similar compounds, e.g. TEPP and malathion, though most are much less toxic than parathion.

Effects

The poison may be absorbed through intact skin, inhaled or ingested. It acts by inhibition of cholinesterase enzymes, so that acetylcholine accumulates at nerve endings, producing stimulation, then paralysis, especially of voluntary muscles. Parathion is extremely toxic and an oral dose of 200 mg may be fatal. Because of this, extensive protective measures are taken, e.g. protective clothing, etc., when the substance is used industrially.

Large overdoses may produce immediate death. Smaller doses cause nausea, vomiting, sweating, abdominal colic, contracted pupils and muscle twitching, followed by convulsions and coma, with muscular paralysis and death from respiratory failure.

Treatment

Contaminated skin must be cleansed and respiration maintained. Specific antidotes are atropine together with PAM (2 pyridine aldoxine methiodide) or pralidoxime chloride.

At autopsy there are no distinctive features of the poison itself but it is commonly supplied in a solvent, such as paraffin, and this may impart a distinctive odour to the tissues.

TOCP (tri-ortho-cresyl phosphate)

Source

An oily liquid, it is used in lubricants and as a plasticiser in industry. Mass outbreaks of poisoning have occurred from contamination of food by containers which previously held the poison. The abortifacient, apiol, may be contaminated by this substance.

Effects

The poison is said to inhibit pseudocholinesterase enzymes with resultant damage to myelin nerve sheaths. Soon after swallowing the poison there is a transient gastric upset. This is followed by a latent period of several days' duration after which pains in the back and legs develop followed by flaccid paralysis of the muscles. The condition may be mistaken for poliomyelitis or some other type of peripheral neuritis.

Carbon monoxide (CO)

Source

Until recently all domestic gas supplies contained CO. Now the introduction of natural gas has made this very rare, and whereas in the past this was the commonest form of suicidal poisoning, it is now rarely seen in these circumstances. However, CO can be produced by incomplete combustion of

Table 27.1.   Toxic effect due to carbon monoxide poisoning.

%HbCO	Symptoms
0–10	No noticeable effects
10–20	Shortness of breath and giddiness may be observed during exercise
20–30	Shortness of breath, giddiness, headache even in the absence of exercise
30–50	Muscular control becomes difficult, resulting in incoordination and staggering Loss of consciousness may be induced by exercise
50–80	Coma, followed by death due to respiratory arrest

any material in a restricted supply of air, for instance by a lighted paraffin heater in an unventilated room. It can also cause death when the fumes from a lit gas fire are returned to the room due to the flue of the fire becoming blocked.

Effects

The gas is absorbed rapidly through the lungs into the blood where it is taken up by haemoglobin in preference to oxygen, producing carboxyhaemoglobin. As this process continues, less and less haemoglobin remains available to transport oxygen, and death results from anoxia (Table 27.1).

Lethal dose

Conversion of more than 50% of the haemoglobin to carboxyhaemoglobin will cause death. In the elderly, or in persons suffering from some serious disease, 30% to 40% conversion may be fatal.

The time taken to die will obviously depend on the concentration of gas inhaled. Thus if pure carbon monoxide is absorbed, as in laboratory accidents, two breaths will absorb sufficient gas to prove fatal. In accidents involving incomplete combustion, with the slower accumulation of carbon monoxide in an unventilated room, death may take much longer to occur.

Signs of poisoning

Cerebral anoxia will cause coma, possibly preceded by convulsions. The carboxyhaemoglobin has a characteristic bright pink colour, which can be seen in the nail beds, the lips, etc. At autopsy the hypostasis, and the internal organs will have the same colour.

Laboratory tests

Carboxyhaemoglobin has a characteristic spectrum by which it can be identified. The amount present in the blood can be determined either by use of a Hartridge reversion spectroscope, or more accurately by gas chromatography.

Treatment

This consists of removing the victim from the contaminated atmosphere, and administering oxygen and assisting respiration if the person is severely poisoned. The anoxia may cause myocardial damage, so that complete rest is necessary for several days. Cerebral anoxia may lead to neurological sequelae. Adminstration of oxygen under raised pressure may increase the removal of carbon monoxide and in some centres hyperbaric oxygen chambers are available for this treatment.

Chlorine (Cl₂)

Although principally an industrial hazard, poisoning has occasionally occurred in domestic circumstances by liberation of chlorine from lavatory cleansers.

The gas produces inflammation of the lungs and pulmonary oedema, and if the victim survives pulmonary fibrosis may result.

Phosgene (COCl₂)

In addition to industrial sources, it may be produced from the action of heat on carbon tetrachloride and trichlorethylene, and thus can be a hazard of the use of some fire extinguishers in confined spaces.

Initial irritation of the respiratory tract, with coughing and choking, is followed, after a latent interval of a few hours, by intense pulmonary oedema. Characteristically at autopsy there is little inflammation of bronchial mucous membrane, in spite of the pulmonary oedema, a finding which distinguishes poisoning by this substance from the effects of chlorine.

Hydrogen sulphide (H₂S)

This gas is produced by putrefaction and so may be found in sewers and tunnels, as well as being produced by various processes in the chemical industry.

The concentrated gas produces fatal poisoning within a few minutes, and lower concentration may cause prolonged unconsciousness, due to cerebral depression.

Sulphur dioxide (SO₂)

Responsible for much of the effects of polluted city air on those with respiratory trouble, it may in high concentration cause severe oedema of the larynx or bronchospasm. Being used at high temperatures in some industrial processes, it may cause burns, which have a characteristic appearance due to fixation instead of charring of the tissues.

Carbon disulphide (CS₂)

Used in many industrial processes. In high concentration it causes cerebral depression and coma, and may lead to respiratory failure. Chronic poisoning with cerebral symptoms, Parkinsonism, chorea, peripheral neuritis, may occur.

Nitrous fumes (NO$_2$ and N$_2$O$_4$)

Hazards of industry, and of laboratory accidents and fires, these red brown irritating fumes produce initial coughing, followed by a latent interval, during which the patient appears to have recovered. However this interval is followed by the development of intense pulmonary oedema. Therefore it is dangerous to send home a person who has recently been exposed to these fumes, even if he appears well. He should be kept under observation for 24 hours, until the danger of pulmonary oedema has passed.

Carbon dioxide (CO$_2$)

The effects of CO$_2$ retention in various diseases and in anaesthesia are well known. Pure CO$_2$ may cause immediate collapse and death, and is a hazard of coal-mining. It may also accumulate in wells, manholes, etc., and cause the sudden death of workmen, often with further deaths among would-be rescuers.

Arsine

See section on arsenic, p. 208.

Phosphine (PH$_3$)

Smells like rotting fish, and is produced in various processes in the chemical industry. A highly toxic gas, it produces the symptoms of cholinesterase inhibition, resembling poisoning by parathion (p. 199) i.e. salivation, sweating, colic, diarrhoea, convulsions, coma, with pinpoint pupils, and death from respiratory depression.

Hydrogen cyanide

See section on cyanide, p. 198.

Methyl bromide (CH$_3$Br)

Used in fire extinguishers and as an insecticide. Very dangerous when used in confined spaces. Symptoms of poisoning are likely to be delayed for several hours, and then commence with gastric upset. The action on the central nervous system produces symptoms resembling mild intoxication, ataxia, diplopia, etc., which are followed by convulsions and pulmonary oedema. Renal tubular necrosis may develop.

Laboratory determination of the blood bromine level may confirm the diagnosis.

There is no antidote, treatment being by symptomatic measures.

Carbon tetrachloride (CCl₄)

Used principally as a fire extinguisher or dry-cleaning agent, and as such it is found in many homes.

Poisoning can be due to inhalation of fumes, as when using a fire extinguisher, or cleaning clothes in a confined space, or by accidental ingestion. Addiction to the fumes may occur, even in children. Coincident ingestion of alcohol increases the toxic effect of the poison.

Inhalation may produce rapid anaesthesia and death within a few minutes. Evidence of poisoning at autopsy is slight, but the organs usually have an odour of carbon tetrachloride, notably the brain, but this may be fleeting, and easily overlooked.

Ingestion of the poison causes initial gastric upset, followed by a latent period of a day or so, after which liver necrosis and renal tubular necrosis develop.

When used as a fire extinguisher, phosgene may be produced (see p. 202).

Tetrachlorethane (CHCl₂)₂

This solvent has many industrial uses. If swallowed accidentally or with suicidal intent it produces cerebral depression and, after a few hours, respiratory failure. Prolonged inhalation, as in industry, may cause fatty degeneration and necrosis of the liver.

Trichlorethylene—trilene (C₂HCl₃)

Well-known as an anaesthetic agent, and also having industrial uses, addiction to the vapour can occur among anaesthetists or workmen. Death has resulted in industry or among addicts from anaesthesia with cerebral and respiratory depression.

Methylene chloride

This substance is used as a paint stripper, and it has been found that after absorption it is metabolised to form carbon monoxide. People exposed to it may develop signs of carbon monoxide poisoning.

Chapter 28
Uncommon Poisons

Quinine

This is freely available as tablets, and as a constituent of tonic mixtures. It may be used as an abortifacient

It is a gastric irritant, causing nausea and vomiting, which is rapidly absorbed. It acts as a cerebral depressant, with particular action on cranial nerves. Thus early signs are headache, tinnitus and blurred vision followed by convulsions and coma. If the patient recovers consciousness he or she may be permanently blind, or deaf, or both. Haemolysis and haemoglobinuria may also occur.

Death may occur from respiratory paralysis during coma, or later from anuria due to blockage of renal tubules by the products of haemolysis.

Treatment consists of gastric lavage and symptomatic measures are required. Blindness can be prevented in some cases by treatment designed to dilate the retinal vessels, such as stellate ganglion blockage, or the use of drugs such as amyl nitrite or nicotinic acid. Forced acid diuresis has been successful on some occasions. However treatment may be required for haemolysis or renal damage.

Chloroquine, which is used as an anti-malarial drug, and in skin diseases, and which may also be used as an abortifacient, may, in overdosage, produce collapse, and death within a short time from sudden cardiac arrest.

Antihistamines

Source

Obtainable as tablets and capsules for use in allergic states and for the prevention of travel sickness.

There are no restrictions on sale, therefore freely available, and particularly dangerous for small children.

Effects

In adults the drugs exert a sedative effect which may be dangerous if the drugs are taken by drivers of motor vehicles, etc. Overdosage will cause the prompt onset of coma, with respiratory depression.

In children, poisoning may produce cerebral excitation with restlessness and muscle twitching progressing to convulsions, followed by coma with respiratory depression and cerebral oedema.

Treatment

Gastric lavage is required together with symptomatic measures, notably the parenteral use of diazepam to control convulsions.

Strychnine

Source

Derived from the seeds of an Indian tree. There are various injections and mixtures containing the salts, hydrochloride, nitrate and sulphate. It was used to effect homicidal poisoning in the nineteenth century, but is nowadays only likely to be encountered in circumstances of accidental poisoning from overdoses of various tonic mixtures which contain strychnine, or from vermin poisons (e.g. for poisoning of moles on golf courses).

Effects

It causes stimulation of the CNS, especially the spinal cord, with exaggeration of reflex arcs. The fatal dose is about 60 mg. Effects commence within about 15 minutes of absorption, and are first apparent as twitching of muscles and the complaint of a feeling of stiffness. This is soon followed by a generalised convulsion, affecting all voluntary muscles of the body. Contraction of the back extensors produces opisthotonus, the hands are clenched, the face distorted into a 'grin'. Spasm of intercostal and diaphragmatic muscles causes respiratory paralysis and cyanosis. Consciousness is retained and intense pain experienced. After about 1 minute the spasm relaxes, and is replaced by exhaustion and respiratory depression. Death may occur after two or more fits. There are no characteristic signs on the body after death, or detectable at autopsy. Differential diagnosis from tetanus may be difficult, but the latter usually has a more insidious onset, a history of injury, affects jaw muscles particularly, and muscles remain tense between spasms.

Treatment

The urgent need is to control the muscle spasms by the use of sedatives such as a barbiturate given intravenously or Valium, or by anaesthesia, and by muscle relaxants such as curare or gallamine.

Once such control has been achieved it may be necessary to maintain respiration artificially. The stomach should be washed out, using a dilute (1/2000) solution of potassium permanganate.

Atropine

Source

Accidental poisoning may occur from medicines containing atropine, e.g.

from liniments or eye-drops. Children may eat the berries of deadly nightshade (*Atropa belladonna*). Sufficient of the drug may be absorbed from the installation of eye-drops to produce bizarre symptoms on occasion.

Effects

Produces CNS stimulation and parasympathetic post-ganglionic blockage. The following mnemonic may be useful:

1 Hot as a hare—pyrexia of 1–6°F.

2 Blind as a bat—dilated fixed pupils, no near focus, and temporary blindness.

3 Dry as a bone—suppression of salivation, as well as other secretions.

4 Red as a beetroot—vasodilatation and scarlatiniform erythema.

5 Daft as a brush—restless and agitated, hallucinations, delirium, inco-ordinated staggering gait, and incoherent speech.

The lethal dose is about 100–150 mg for adults.

Treatment

If the poison was ingested gastric lavage is indicated, though if children have eaten berries, then emesis may be preferable as the berries will probably not pass through the stomach tube. The physiological antidote is the parasym-pathomimetic drug, i.e. physostigmine salicylate. In addition general measures should be employed, notably sedation, control of pyrexia, and possibly bladder catheterisation for retention of urine.

At autopsy evidence of poisoning is unlikely unless, in a child, berries are found in the stomach.

Nicotine

Source

This is mainly found as insecticide solutions which may contain up to 98% of nicotine, but accidental poisoning can occur, especially in children, from swallowing tobacco or the tarry fluid which accumulates in pipes. The solution can be absorbed through intact skin, e.g. from contaminated clothing.

Effects

The substance behaves like curare in that it paralyses voluntary muscles, particularly the muscles of respiration, and blocks the nicotinic actions of the sympathetic and parasympathetic ganglia. Symptoms of poisoning may be an exaggeration of the effects of heavy smoking, e.g. nausea and vomiting, cold sweats, faintness and dizziness, and these may be followed by convulsions or coma, and respiratory paralysis.

If large doses are taken in a suicidal attempt, however, the victim is likely to collapse and die almost immediately from respiratory paralysis. A fatal dose may be about 60 mg.

Chronic poisoning may produce Buerger's disease (thromboangiitis obliterans) or tobacco amblyopia.

Treatment

Any contaminated clothing must be removed at once, and skin washed.

Ingested poison may be removed by gastric lavage with dilute potassium permanganate.

Since the main lethal effect of nicotine is respiratory paralysis, principally of the muscles, but in heavy doses of the medulla also, and since the substance is rapidly destroyed in the body, artificial respiration until the effects of the poison have worn off is the most important measure in saving life.

At autopsy the stomach may be stained brown and smell of stale tobacco.

Aconite

Source

This is derived from the plant *Aconitium napellus* or monkshood, which is grown in many English gardens. It is a component of some medicines, notably liniment ABC.

Effects

The poison is extremely dangerous, 2 mg of the active principle, aconitine, being said to constitute a fatal dose. The action of the alkaloid is on nerve endings, and, to a lesser extent, on the brain.

If swallowed there is an initial tingling of the lips and mouth, followed by vomiting and dysphagia. A sensation of coldness extends over the body with progressive muscular paralysis, the pulse rate is slowed and death results from respiratory paralysis.

Conium (hemlock)

Derived from the hemlock plant, found throughout Britain. The alkaloid coniine has an action resembling that of curare, with progressive motor paralysis extending upwards from the extremities until death results from respiratory paralysis. The drug was used to poison Socrates. Treatment is by artificial respiration, oxygen, and analeptics.

Arsenic

Source

The most notorious of the homicidal poisons, restrictions ensure nowadays that the principal source of the poison is in industry, such as in glass manufacture, sheep dips, fruit sprays, etc. Traces occur naturally in some soils, well waters, shellfish, etc. Mass poisonings have occurred occasionally from accidental contamination of food. The various forms of arsenic which cause poisoning are arsenious oxide, various arsenites and sulphites of arsenic, arsine gas and organic arsenicals.

The lethal dose of arsenious oxide is about 120 mg. The principal effects of poisoning are produced by combination of the poison with sulphydryl groups of enzymes.

Symptoms

1 Ingested poison:

(a) *Fulminating*—massive doses may cause shock with peripheral vascular collapse and death may occur in 1–2 hours. This form of poisoning is rare.

(b) *Acute*—the typical effects of irritant poisoning are produced, i.e. pain, vomiting, diarrhoea, circulatory failure. Death may occur in 12–36 hours.

(c) *Chronic*—when taken in small doses over a period of weeks or months. General debility, weight loss, chronic gastrointestinal disturbance, mental irritability, loss of hair, 'rain-drop' pigmentation of the skin and hyperkeratosis of palms and soles, and peripheral neuritis.

2 Inhaled poison. Arsine gas (AsH_3) is an industrial hazard. It produces massive haemolysis. Death may occur at once, or within a few days, due to renal damage resulting principally from the effects of haemolysis.

3 Injected poison. Organic arsenicals, e.g. used in treatment of syphilis, have produced sudden collapse and death. The overuse of pessaries containing arsenic, e.g. for trichomonas, has also caused poisoning.

Laboratory tests

Arsenic may be found in the stomach contents in cases of acute poisoning; and in the blood and urine, faeces, and hair in cases of chronic poisoning.

After burial arsenic may remain detectable in the organs for many months and the body tends to be abnormally well preserved. Care must be taken to exclude the possibility of contamination of the body by arsenic derived from the soil of the grave before arriving at the conclusion that death was due to poisoning.

Treatment

In acute cases use gastric lavage. If available ferric hydroxide will precipitate any poison remaining in the stomach. The specific antidote BAL (British anti-lewisite), which has greater affinity than the sulphydryl groups of the enzymes for arsenic. It should be given as early as possible.

In chronic poisoning the patient must be removed from the source of the poisoning; in other words, if homicidal poisoning is suspected, the patient should be admitted to hospital. Treatment with BAL must be instituted.

Antimony

This substance is similar in many respects to arsenic. It is used in tropical medicine, and in industry. The compounds mainly responsible for poisoning are potassium antimony tartrate (tartar emetic) and antimony chloride. It has been used for homicide, but toxic effects are nowadays likely to be the result of accidental ingestion. Group poisonings have occurred from contamination of food and drink by traces of antimony in the enamel of utensils. It does not occur naturally in soil.

The effects are similar to those of arsenic, i.e. blockage of sulphydryl groups. Vomiting is particularly pronounced (hence tartar emetic). Antimony may damage the heart muscle and cause bradycardia or sudden heart failure, especially when given intravenously as in the treatment of tropical diseases.

Treatment is by gastric lavage and BAL.

Phosphorus

When phosphorus was a constituent of rat poisons, and therefore readily available to the public, cases of poisoning were not infrequent in this country. Now its only source is likely to be in industry. There are two forms of phosphorus, the yellow, which is poisonous, and the red which is innocuous.

Effects

The poison has a garlic odour and taste, and is unlikely to be taken accidentally. It can produce three forms of poisoning:

1   Fulminating. Death occurs in a few hours, and the principal features are of peripheral vascular collapse.

2   Acute. The most common form. Initial symptoms are of irritant poison, burning pain, vomiting, severe thirst. The vomit may be luminous. These symptoms last for up to 48 hours. Then for 1 or 2 days there is a remission of symptoms. Finally signs of liver damage develop, with enlargement of the liver, jaundice, multiple haemorrhages, and hepatic coma.

3   Chronic. This form of poisoning is rare, but has occurred in workers handling phosphorus, poisoning being from the fumes. The principal effect is necrosis of the bones of the jaw, together with chronic gastrointestinal disturbances and liver damage.

Treatment

Gastric lavage with dilute potassium permanganate to oxidise the phosphorus or copper sulphate. General measures to treat shock, liver failure, or renal failure.

Copper sulphate will neutralise the phosphorus and a copper sulphate-soap mixture is useful in the treatment of phosphorus burns on the skin, which are deep and devitalising.

At the autopsy of a person who has died in the early stages of poisoning, signs of acute gastrointestinal irritation with luminous garlic-smelling intestinal contents are indicative of the poison. If the victim has survived for a few days, jaundice with acute fatty changes or necrosis of the liver and fatty degeneration of other organs, together with multiple haemorrhages within the body, are likely to be found. When taking samples it must be remembered that elemental phosphorus will be rapidly oxidised if the material is exposed to air for any time and so samples must be put into sealed containers as soon as possible. The stomach and bowel are better left unopened.

DNOC (di-nitro-ortho-cresol)

Principally used as weedkiller and insecticide. At one time it had a therapeutic use in the treatment of obesity.

Absorption can be through the skin, as well as by injection and inhalation, so that persons spraying crops are at risk if they do not wear protective clothing.

The action of the poison is to produce a considerable increase of the basal metabolic rate. Initial feelings of unusual well-being are followed by fatigue, insomnia, thirst and sweating, and loss of weight. Raised respiration rate and hyperpyrexia are followed by convulsions, coma and death.

There is no specific antidote. Any poison left on the skin must be removed; general measures will be required, in particular, sedation which should be with chlorpromazine, and reduction of pyrexia.

Chapter 29
Poisoning in Childhood

Poisoning of children is particularly important since they are more liable to suffer from accidental poisoning than adults, being prone to experiment with tastes and to put things in their mouths, and to be attracted by brightly coloured pills which resemble sweets. It has been suggested that children are particularly liable to suffer accidents such as poisoning at times of stress in the family in general.

The principle of diagnosis and treatment of poisoning in childhood is on the same general lines as adults, and no attempt is made, therefore, in this book to deal with the particular aspects of medical treatment of children, which are the province of paediatrics. Suffice it to say that poisoning should always be considered as a possible cause of sudden illness in a child, though the differentiation of such a condition from the early symptoms of an acute infection may be difficult.

Since accidental poisoning in children is so often preventable, doctors should endeavour whenever possible to ensure that parents lock medicines and poisons in safe places, out of the reach of children, and to avoid the accumulation in the house of large amounts of unused medicines.

Recent legislation has recognised the importance of reducing the availability of medicines to children. The Medicines (Child Safety) Regulations 1975 stipulate that children's aspirin and paracetamol preparations are to be sold or supplied only in child-proof containers and only when coloured white. Not more than 24 tablets are to be available in a container. Increasing use is now made of child-proof containers with special caps or with press-out foil packaging of tablets to prevent the easy acquisition of them by children.

The substances commonly causing poisoning in children are mostly those which are freely available and which also cause adult poisoning. These have been mentioned in detail in the preceding pages. A few substances however are likely to be especially consumed by children, or have peculiar dangers for them, and these will be described in this chapter.

The principal substances causing poisoning in children are:
1 Salicylates.
2 Tranquillisers.
3 Iron preparations.
4 Paracetamol.
5 Benzodiazepines.

Others of importance, though less commonly responsible for poisoning are:

6 Barbiturates.

7 Strychnine.

8 Antihistamines.

9 Paraffin.

10 Lead.

11 Digitalis.

12 Atropine.

13 Paraquat.

14 Borax.

Salicylates (see p. 182)

Aspirin tablets or methyl salicylate liniment are equally dangerous. Thus 1 teaspoon of the liniment contains 3 g of salicylate.

Poisoning may occur from accidental consumption of the ubiquitous aspirin tablets, but it may also occur from the excessive administration by parents of aspirin to children who are ill from some cause, such as a mild infection or from teething. The classical symptoms, e.g. dyspnoea, will be seen and the condition may be mistaken for pneumonia. Children are much more likely to die from salicylate poisoning than are adults.

Antidepressants (see p. 181)

Reported cases have shown ataxia, nystagmus, athetoid movements and epileptiform convulsions, together with irregularities of the heart due to interference with the mechanism of conduction and with the risk of cardiac arrest.

Iron preparations

These are peculiarly dangerous for children, and the brightly coloured tablets may closely resemble sweets. A fatal dose may be about 1 g (i.e. 5–6 tablets).

Symptoms may occur in three stages:

1 Stage of gastrointestinal irritation lasting about 6 hours, with abdominal pain, vomiting and shock due to necrotising effect of iron on the bowel mucosa.

2 Latent period, lasting about 24 hours, during which time the child appears to be recovering, though toxic products are being formed within the body.

3 Relapse due to development of acidosis or the toxic effect of free iron in the circulation. There may be convulsions or coma, with liver damage, and haemorrhages. Death may occur in either the first or third stage.

Treatment is by emesis to remove the tablets, or gastric lavage with sodium bicarbonate solution to precipitate the iron in the stomach. The specific antidote is desferrioxamine, some being instilled into the stomach and some given by intravenous infusion.

Antihistamines

Children are more likely to be poisoned by these drugs than are adults, since only a small amount may constitute a toxic dose, and because antihistamine preparations are readily available in many homes being used as remedies for travel sickness or hay-fever.

The principal symptoms in children are likely to be of cerebral irritation with ataxia and delirium, followed by convulsions. Death may occur from respiratory depression.

Borax

This has been a common household substance used in the care of children for many years, in the form of dusting powders or boracic lotion. The BMA has (1965) advised doctors not to prescribe boracic compounds and the Poisons Board has recommended that manufacturers should stop making preparations containing boric acid and borates for infants. They can, however, still be found in preparations obtained abroad.

Borax can be absorbed by ingestion, or through broken skin (e.g. a nappy-rash) but not through intact skin.

Symptoms

1   Gastrointestinal irritation—vomiting, diarrhoea, shock. Rash—red and beefy.
2   Cerebral symptoms—delirium, convulsions and coma with neck retraction (meningeal irritation).
3   Renal symptoms—oliguria and anuria.

The coincidence of gastrointestinal and meningeal symptoms in a child with a pronounced skin rash should always suggest the possibility of borax poisoning.

Lead

Children are especially at risk from this particular substance. Sources of poisoning may be from toys containing lead, lead paints, cosmetics, etc.

Affected children will at first be listless, pale, and anaemic. However, unlike adults suffering from lead poisoning, the symptoms are likely to progress to the development of behaviour disturbances and restlessness, followed by encephalopathy, which may be fatal or cause residual mental retardation. Some cases of mental deficiency have been found to be associated with high levels of lead in the body.

Camphor

Poisoning is likely to be by the liniment, camphorated oil. Camphor was popular in medicine at one time as an analeptic, and so the symptoms of overdosage are of cerebral irritation, headache, restlessness and confusion, muscle twitching and convulsions. Poisoning is rarely fatal but may cause death from respiratory failure. A teaspoonful of the liniment may prove fatal to an infant.

Digitalis

From swallowing adults' pills or medicines. The effects of the poison are to produce nausea and vomiting, followed by cardiac disturbances, such as bradycardia, heart block, as in overdosage in adults. Death from heart failure is rare.

Poisonous plants

Many common plants are poisonous and children are especially liable to eat their berries or chew their leaves. Some plants have already been mentioned—monkshood (aconite, p. 208), hemlock (*Conium*, p. 208), foxglove (*Digitalis*, p. 215), deadly nightshade (atropine, p. 206). Other plants commonly found which can produce poisoning, usually with gastro-intestinal irritation as the principal feature, are laburnum, broom, privet, *Daphne mezereum*, cyclamen, hawthorn, horsechestnut.

Similar danger may arise from toadstools. The most dangerous is *Amanita phalloides*, the death cap. Effects are delayed for several hours, when vomiting, abdominal pain and diarrhoea commence and become severe, with dehydration and shock. After 3 or 4 days liver or renal failure is likely to develop, with coma and death.

Other mushrooms, e.g. *Amanita muscaria*, may produce symptoms suggesting alcoholic intoxication, with salivation, nausea and vomiting, hallucinations and convulsions.

Chapter 30
Drug Addiction

At one time a minor problem in this country, with addiction confined to the morphine group of drugs and with addicts only numbered in a few hundreds, the situation has altered rapidly in recent years. It is considered that there are nowadays large numbers of people addicted to drugs of many different types, sedatives, stimulants, etc., as well as the narcotics, and such addiction is increasingly found among young people, even schoolchildren.

People who become drug addicts usually need much money to obtain supplies of the drug, but are incapable of working and so are likely to turn to crime, prostitution or robbery. The intoxicating or hallucinogenic effects of some drugs may result in crimes of violence.

A laudable attempt to deal with the problem of drug abuse has been the enactment of the Misuse of Drugs Act 1971 with its several more recent regulations. Under the provisions of this statute, a doctor is required to notify to the appropriate authority particulars of any person who he suspects is addicted to drugs. He may not supply drugs to such persons except under licence from the Home Secretary, and contravention of regulations made under the provisions of the Act may result in the doctor being prohibited from supplying such drugs of addiction. Alleged contravention of regulations by doctors may be considered by special tribunals. For further details see Chapter 9.

Certain groups of drugs are especially prone to produce addiction, and this danger must be borne in mind when prescribing such drugs for a patient.

Morphine group

These were the original and are the best-known drugs of addiction, principally opium, morphine, pethedine, heroin, methadone, etc. They produce intense craving and severe withdrawal symptoms, and heroin especially is associated with rapid physical and mental degeneration. Treatment of a patient by one of these drugs for more than 2 weeks is liable to produce addiction. The drugs are frequently self-administered intravenously, with lack of sterile precautions, and so addicts may be recognised by thrombosis of superficial veins and multiple small abscesses at injection sites on arms and legs. Apart from the general physical and moral effects of addiction, the victims are also at risk of overdose of the drug, septicaemia and serum hepatitis. The drugs can be detected in the urine, as can most of the other drugs of abuse, except some of the hallucinogens.

Poisoning by morphine produces a deep coma, with contracted 'pinpoint' pupils, very slow respiration (about 6/minute), warm sweating skin, and hypotension. Excretion of urine is diminished, and reflexes depressed.

With large doses death may occur from respiratory depression within an hour, but with smaller amounts coma is likely to be prolonged with the risk of hypostatic pneumonia occurring. The lethal dose is about 180 mg but children are disproportionately sensitive to the drug, for their body size.

Treatment consists of maintenance of respiration, often by artificial means, and the injection of the specific antagonist, naloxone hydrochloride 0.4 mg intravenously or intramuscularly. Recovery should be rapid. Morphine is mainly excreted in the urine and therefore the bladder should be catheterised.

Heroin, methadone, and omnopon and various compounds of morphine such as chlorodine can produce a similar picture.

Pethedine has a relatively slight hypnotic effect compared to morphine but tends to produce cerebral excitation. An overdose will initially have similar effects to that of atropine or cocaine, i.e. flushed face with dilated pupils, dry mouth, tachycardia, pyrexia, vomiting, excitement, tremors and convulsions. If pethidine is combined with a phenothiazine drug alarming or fatal collapse may occur.

Cocaine group

These produce intense craving for the drug, but no physical withdrawal symptoms. Cocaine may be taken as snuff ('snorting snow') or it may be injected either by itself or in combination with other drugs such as benzodiazepines. A new form of cocaine known as 'crack', so named because of its fissure-like surface after it has been chemically activated and heated, is considerably more addictive and markedly heightens the excitement and other sensations. It may result in perforation of the nasal septum if it is abused over a long period. The addict is likely to show excitement, and will probably experience 'formication', a sensation as of insects crawling under the skin. There may in fact be dermatitis with skin ulcers.

Poisoning by a large dose causes cerebral stimulation with excitement and confusion, progressing to convulsions which are followed by coma, with respiratory depression and death. Treatment of an overdose consists of control of excitement by short-acting barbiturates or diazepam, and maintenance of respiration.

Cannabis group

Cannabis does not usually cause physical deterioration or withdrawal symptoms, and addiction does not produce social degeneration caused by the other substances, but it is dangerous because it may act as an introduction for young people to the other forms of addiction. Its symptoms are rather similar to alcoholic intoxication, producing distortion of perception, a sense of unreality, and hallucinations, and sexual excitement. Larger amounts cause dizziness and ataxia, delirium, and deep sleep. It is said to have been the drug used by the original sect of Assassins. The drug is usually taken by inhalation from cigarettes ('reefers'). Liquid preparations or heated resin (the form in which the cannabis is usually smuggled into this country), are mixed with tobacco before the cigarette is rolled. The smell of burning cannabis is characteristic. There is some evidence to suggest that cannabis can produce long-term damage to the brain.

Barbiturate group

Any barbiturate or any sedative drug can produce addiction, the patient taking progressively larger amounts, much greater than the therapeutic dose. There may be severe withdrawal symptoms. Consumption of such a sedative for more than 4 weeks may produce addiction. These drugs may be taken together with alcohol, or with stimulant drugs, and in such circumstances may produce sudden and unexpected death. Though usually taken orally, they may be administered intravenously, with similar dangers to those described under morphine above. The starch excipient of the capsules may produce micro-emboli of the lungs, detectable at autopsy. This form of addiction may affect middle-aged people, where drug addiction is not anticipated, and cause dangers when the addict becomes suddenly deprived of his regular doses, as for instance on acute admission to hospital for illness, when withdrawal symptoms may result.

Amphetamine group

These drugs are particularly liable to be taken by young people for their stimulant action, though voluntary control of prescribing by doctors and pharmacists has considerably reduced the problem. However in some countries illicit 'factories' have produced quantities of amphetamines in simple processes in ordinary rooms.

Addicts may be restless, or experience paranoid hallucinations, have a dry mouth and ulceration of the oral mucosa and may develop sleeplessness, maniacal behaviour or even hyperpyrexia. Overdosage may cause cerebral excitation with continuous purposeless physical activity, raised blood pressure, and hyperpyrexia. Hallucinations and convulsions may progress to exhaustion and coma with respiratory paralysis. Treatment is sedation to control the cerebral excitement by chlorpromazine or barbiturates, and symptomatic measures to reduce hyperpyrexia.

Hallucinogenic group

Although such drugs as LSD (lysergic acid diethylamide), mescaline, etc., are not yet proved to produce true addiction, illegal supply has allowed them to reach the groups of society who are particularly liable to drug addiction. Special cults have grown up around their use. They produce profound alterations in perception ('going on a trip') and have been held to be valuable in stimulating artistic creation, with extraordinary conceptions of colour and form. This may have been responsible for several deaths, since they produce hallucinations in the recipients, with such impressions as that they can fly, dive through brick walls, etc. They can produce terrifying psychotic episodes as well—'a bad trip'. Such episodes may occur many months after the last dose of LSD was taken and are apparently triggered off by some apparently unrelated stimulus. Many of the drugs are produced in illegal laboratories, and as the dose is very small, can be supplied in such vehicles as small pieces of paper impregnated with tiny drops of the solution. Single tablets may be brightly coloured and very small; 'microdots'. Only a few micrograms of the drug are necessary to produce the desired effects.

Volatile substances

An increasingly common problem is the development of addiction to the various volatile agents. These range from ether and carbon tetrachloride, to toluene-based contact adhesives to cigarette lighter fuel and even some forms of fire extinguishers. Schoolchildren have been found to be especially prone to this practice. There is danger from many of the agents of long-term damage to liver or kidneys. An acute overdose may produce fatal poisoning, like an anaesthetic fatality, but often inhalation of the volatile substances results in regurgitation of vomitus and inhalation into the air passages. In a few cases there is strong evidence that the sudden death is caused by a direct excitation of the heart muscle by the solvent. Addicts often inhale the volatile agent on a piece of cloth or paper held inside a plastic bag placed over the head, and this practice is obviously especially dangerous. The practice of inhalation of such agents may result in sores of the skin around the nose.

Treatment of drug addiction

Medical practitioners should always be on their guard to recognise addicts or potential addicts, to be cautious in prescribing any of the drugs known to produce addiction, and to ensure that large supplies of drugs are not available to patient's homes to be passed onto those without authority to receive them. The requirements of the Misuse of Drugs Act 1971 must be observed precisely, not least because failure to do so will render the doctor liable to prosecution.

Treatment of drug addiction should only be carried out by medical practitioners having special experience and facilities, e.g. in mental hospitals, and such treatment should not be undertaken lightly. Centres have been set up by the government in an attempt to answer the problem of treatment. The prevention and cure of drug addiction is as serious a problem as prevention of the major infectious diseases, because of its terrible destructive effect on the physical well-being of the patients, and their families, and on their mental states.

Drug addiction does not usually affect psychologically normal people but is liable to be found in those already suffering from some mental disorder or defect of personality, especially inadequacies. Therefore treatment consists as much of psychiatric treatment for the underlying personality disorder as of withdrawal abruptly or gradually, or by substitution, of the drug.

It should be realised that chronic alcoholism can be regarded as a form of drug addiction, and indeed at present poses equally great problems in treatment, and far greater ones in terms of numbers of people affected in our society.

Books for Reference or Further Reading

Burges S. H. (ed) (1978) *The New Police Surgeon: a practical guide to clinical forensic medicine*. Hutchinson, London.

Camps F. E., Robinson A. E. and Lucas B. G. B. (eds) (1976) *Gradwohl's Legal Medicine*, 3rd edn. John Wright, Bristol.

Gresham G. A. (1975) *A Colour Atlas of Forensic Pathology*. Wolfe Medical Books, London.

Knight B. (1987) *Legal Aspects of Medical Practice*, 4th edn. Churchill Livingstone, Edinburgh.

Mant A. K. (1984) *Taylor's Principles and Practice of Forensic Medicine*, 13th edn. J. and A. Churchill Ltd, London.

Mason J. K. (1978) *The Pathology of Violent Injury*. Edward Arnold, London.

Mason J. K. (1983) *Forensic Medicine for Lawyers*, 2nd edn. Butterworth, London.

Matthew H. and Lawton A. A. H. (1975) *Treatment of Common Acute Poisonings*, 3rd edn. Churchill Livingstone, London.

Polson C. J., Gee D. J. and Knight B. (1985) *The Essentials of Forensic Medicine*. Pergamon Press, Oxford.

Polson C. J., Green M. A. and Lee M. R. (1983) *Clinical Toxicology*, 3rd edn. Pitman, London.

Polson C. J. and Marshall T. K. (1975) *Disposal of the Dead*, 3rd edn. English Universities Press Ltd, London.

Proudfoot A. (1982) *Diagnosis and Management of Acute Poisoning*. Blackwell Scientific Publications, Oxford.

Rentoul E. and Smith H. (eds) (1973) *Glaister's Medical Jurisprudence*, 13th edn. Churchill Livingstone, Edinburgh.

Simpson K. and Knight B. (1985) *Forensic Medicine*, 9th edn. Edward Arnold, London.

Taylor J. Leahy (1982) *The Doctor and the Law*, 2nd edn. Pitman Medical and Scientific Publishing Company, London.

Watson A. A. (1989) *Forensic Medicine, A Handbook for Professionals*. Gower Publishing Company, Aldershot.

Index

Notes on specific cases